AF675639

Psychopharmacology and Psychotherapy

Psychopharmacology and Psychotherapy

EDITED BY
Maurice H. Greenhill, M.D.
Alexander Gralnick, M.D.

FP
THE FREE PRESS
A Division of Macmillan Publishing Co., Inc.
NEW YORK
Collier Macmillan Publishers
LONDON

Copyright © 1983 by Maurice H. Greenhill, M.D.
and Alexander Gralnick, M.D.

All rights reserved. No part of this book may be reproduced or transmitted in any form or by any means, electronic or mechanical, including photocopying, recording, or by any information storage and retrieval system, without permission in writing from the Publisher.

The Free Press
A Division of Macmillan Publishing Co., Inc.
866 Third Avenue, New York, N.Y. 10022

Collier Macmillan Canada, Inc.

Printed in the United States of America

printing number

1 2 3 4 5 6 7 8 9 10

Library of Congress Cataloging in Publication Data
Main entry under title:

Psychopharmacology and psychotherapy.

Papers originally presented at a conference in New York City Apr. 11–12, 1980, which was organized by the Albert Einstein College of Medicine and High Point Hospital (Psychiatric) of Port Chester, N.Y.

Includes index.

1. Psychopharmacology—Congresses. 2. Psychotherapy—Congresses. I. Greenhill, Maurice H. II. Gralnick, Alexander. III. Albert Einstein College of Medicine. IV. High Point Hospital. [DNLM: 1. Mental disorders—Drug therapy. 2. Psychotherapy. WM 402 P9753]
RC483.P7775 1983 616.89′14 82-71886

ISBN 0-02-912780-7

These collected papers are dedicated posthumously to Maurice H. Greenhill, M.D. (8/16/09–1/20/81), who planned and organized the meeting at which they were given. He was a sensitive and skillful psychiatrist, a leader in his field, an inspiring teacher, and above all, a role model of the philosophy, methods, and quality of patient care which he advocated.

Contents

Foreword

THE RECENT HISTORY of psychiatry has disclosed a nearly impermeable membrane between those with a psychodynamic view and those with a biological outlook on psychiatric disorders. The dominance of psychodynamic theory and practice during the 1950s and 1960s has only recently been challenged by the signal discoveries of biological researchers and by the demonstration of the efficacy of pharmacotherapy in the treatment of the psychoses. Indeed, the enthusiasm arising from the success of the biological approach now threatens to submerge psychodynamic psychiatry, placing the entire profession at risk of neglecting hard-won, powerful insights into human behavior and illness. Such is man's temperament that he finds it difficult to pledge allegiance to more than one philosophy at a time. To immerse oneself intuitively and empathically in another's thoughts, feelings, and experience seems to preclude a more objective, scientific appraisal of the correlative biological processes, and vice versa. Pascal's observation—that the heart has reasons of which the head knows nothing—is a reciprocal relationship.

A virtue of this volume is that it challenges this conceptual insularity by highlighting a modern therapeutic trend of major importance for the treatment of psychiatric patients and for the future of psychiatry as a profession. Collectively, the chapters in this book stress the need to combine psychotherapeutic and pharmacotherapeutic treatment approaches, and they provide evidence that, for many patients, this combination is more effective than either treatment modality used alone. In so doing, this book follows the lead of a few earlier, pioneering publications, such as the GAP Report of 1975, "Pharmacotherapy and Psychotherapy: Paradoxes, Problems, and Progress," in which several of the authors represented here participated. The acorn planted during the last decade is clearly growing into a sturdy young oak.

Although the individual chapters focus mainly on treatment, their emphasis on the need for a synthesis of biological and psychological concepts has an important bearing on psychiatric observation, theory, and training. Dr. Ostow's discussion, for example, of the need for a detailed observation of the mental states of patients undergoing pharmacotherapy points to an application of psychoanalytic technique that is often overlooked when the focus is on biological treatment. As he demonstrates in graphic clinical vignettes, only through careful, sensitive, and empathic listening to one's patients can one detect the subtle nuances of their mental states as they undergo the subjective experiences brought about by altering their physiology through medication. Such psychological observations provide important clinical data for determining the choice of medication, for monitoring its optimum therapeutic level, and for assessing its effectiveness. In short, one might suggest that the experienced psychoanalyst is in an ideal position to prescribe for his patients, whether the treatment be psychological, biological, or a combination of both.

Psychiatric theory can be similarly enhanced by a judicious marriage of biological and psychological concepts, and the tendency still prevalent among many psychiatrists to think in either/or terms must be tempered by a recognition of the complementarity of the two orientations. The discovery that certain forms of depression or anxiety have significant biological correlates does not necessarily mean that they are entirely "autonomous" in nature and therefore unrelated to psychic conflict; rather, it suggests that certain individuals specially sensitized by their biological constitutions may react with unusual symptomatic severity to psychic conflicts that in another person not so constituted lead to symptoms of lesser, more manageable intensity. The use of medication to control incapacitating symptoms should not preclude psychotherapy aimed at resolving pathogenic conflicts, nor should psychotherapy forfend the simultaneous use of drugs designed to stabilize biological functioning. The broader the psychiatrist's conceptual view of symptom formation, the more flexible and effective his therapeutic approach.

The prescription for such a therapeutic and conceptual flexibility is easy to write. It may be harder to swallow if, as a profession, we cannot break down the barriers that tend to compartmentalize most of us into psychodynamic and biological psychiatrists. The remedy for this conceptual rigidity lies in part in psychiatric training. Medical school has given the psychiatric resident the biological education he needs to become a physician; it is the task of residency training to add the psychodynamic education that will transform him into a physician specializing in psychiatric disorders. But more is required than merely the sequential exposure of psychiatrists-in-training to these two orientations. They must somehow be taught to synthesize the biological and psychodynamic views of psychiatric illness; otherwise, as so often seems to be the case with graduates of modern psychiatric residency programs, they will narrowly pursue one approach without an adequate appreciation of the other.

This is not the place to discuss how the resident's education might help him achieve such a synthesis. Indeed, the specific means for accomplishing it are not now readily apparent, and the task of devising them lies ahead as a major educational challenge. Suffice it to say that, insofar as they have succeeded in weaving biology and psychology into a single fabric, the authors of these chapters provide us with models for emulation. In the long run, the major contribution of this important volume may be its effect on the education of the psychiatrists of the future.

John C. Nemiah, M.D.

Preface

THE TWO PRINCIPAL MODALITIES of treatment in modern psychiatry are psychotherapy and psychopharmacology. Methods and techniques of psychotherapy were well established before the advent of psychopharmacology as it is known today. Many models of psychotherapy precluded or discouraged the use of medication as an adjunct in treatment. So important was the therapist-patient relationship in the methods of psychotherapy that it appeared to be an inviolate rule that there be only one therapist.

During the past two decades, psychopharmacological agents have proven to be so effective in the care of the mentally ill that three new conditions in psychiatric care have emerged: (1) most mental health professionals practicing psychotherapy now use drugs as well in the treatment of their patients; (2) clinical psychopharmacologists, who frequently believe that psychotherapy is a lesser modality, are finding that the interaction between the patient and the physician is still quite a significant factor and that psychosocial influences are not unimportant in the process of treatment with drugs; and (3) the psychiatric patient today often becomes involved with two therapists, one who is the principal psychotherapist (psychiatrist, psychologist, social worker, or nurse) and the other the administrator of medication (general psychiatrist, biological psychiatrist, or clinical psychopharmacologist).

These new conditions have raised many questions, both within the mental health professions and with patients. Discussions of priorities are just emerging. Dualistic thinking is, unfortunately, active, with traditional psychotherapists and conventional psychopharmacologists taking either/or positions on the relative efficacy of their treatment system. Relatively few papers or books on these issues have been published, and, until April 1980, no symposium had been convened to serve both as a forum for biological psychiatrists and psychotherapists and as an occasion for the reporting of investigative work on these subjects.

For these reasons, a symposium entitled "The Interrelationship of Psychotherapy and Psychopharmacology" was organized by the Albert Einstein College of Medicine and High Point Hospital (psychiatric) of Port Chester, New York, under a grant from the Gralnick Foundation. It was held at the Hilton Hotel in New York City on April 11–12, 1980. Speakers invited to present papers were selected from American leaders in the fields of psychotherapy and psychopharmacology who were most expert and actively concerned in the issues of such conjoint therapy as adjudged by their research work, writings, and stated positions. They came from the fields of general psychiatry, psychoanalysis, psychology, social work, and biological psychiatry.

The thesis of the conference was stated as follows:

> Advances in biological psychiatry and psychopharmacology do not indicate reduction in the importance of interpersonal relations in the lives of patients or of psychotherapy in the treatment of psychiatric disorders. What is required is change in the conceptualization of the interrelationship of psychotherapy and psychopharmacology and restructuring of methods of combining these modalities of treatment. This symposium will address these issues, particularly the current tendencies to dualistic thinking and the dynamics of combined therapy. We will also explore the attitudes of biological psychiatrists toward psychotherapy and the neuroscience orientation of psychoanalysts. We will review the problems of multiple therapists in conjoint therapy by mental health professionals and clinical psychopharmacologists.

The topic was considered so timely and important to American psychiatry, psychology, social work, and nursing—and the response to the symposium was so enthusiastic—that we have edited their papers and brought them together in this book.

About the Contributors

Michael J. Goldstein received his Ph.D. in clinical psychology from the University of Washington in 1957. Since then his affiliation has been with the University of California, Los Angeles. He has been a Fulbright research Professor at the University of Copenhagen and has served as a member of numerous national advisory committees. The author of four books and over sixty articles, he has served on the editorial boards of various journals.

Frederick K. Goodwin, M.D., is the Director of the NIMH Intramural Research Program. A 1963 graduate of St. Louis University School of Medicine, he has authored over 300 publications, including a major book on manic depressive illness (with Dr. Kay Jamison). He is one of five psychiatrists on the *Current Contents* list of the most frequently cited authors and has received several awards.

Alexander Gralnick, M.D., is a Medical Director of High Point Hospital, a psychiatric institution which he founded in 1951; he is

Associate Clinical Professor of Psychiatry at New York Medical College. He has authored more than seventy-five papers and is the editor and main contributor of two books, *The Psychiatric Hospital as a Therapeutic Instrument* and *Humanizing the Psychiatric Hospital.*

Roy R. Grinker, Sr., M.D., is Professor Emeritus of Psychiatry at the University of Chicago and Michael Reese Hospital. He is the author of eighteen books and 265 journal articles and chapters in various books. Originally a neurologist, he then became a psychiatrist and psychologist. He was analyzed by Sigmund Freud in Vienna and has received many awards and citations.

Gerard E. Hogarty, M.S.W., is Associate Professor of Psychiatry and Director of Schizophrenia Research, Western Psychiatric Institute and Clinic, University of Pittsburgh School of Medicine. Previously he was Chief, Social Science Research, Friends Medical Science Research Center, Baltimore, Maryland and Director NIMH Collaborative Outpatient Studies in Schizophrenia. He has published extensively.

Kay Jamison, Ph.D., is Associate Professor at the University of California, Los Angeles, from which she received her doctorate. In addition, she is director of the Affective Disorders Clinic at the University of California, Los Angeles. Among her publications is a major book on manic depressive illnesses in collaboration with Frederick Goodwin.

Donald F. Klein, M.D., is Director of Psychiatric Research at the New York State Psychiatric Institute and Professor of Psychiatry, College of Physicians & Surgeons of Columbia University, New York. He is a coauthor of several well-known textbooks on psychopharmacology and psychiatric diagnosis and has written (with Paul Wender, M.D.) a book for the general public, *Mind Mood & Medicine: A Guide to the New Biopsychiatry.*

Gerald L. Klerman, M.D. (New York University), is on the Psychiatry Service of the Massachusetts General Hospital, where he is Director of the Stanley Cobb Laboratories for Research and George Harrington Professor of Psychiatry at Harvard Medical School and Director of the Harvard Program in Psychiatric Epidemiology. He has also taught at Yale University. Formerly, he served as Administrator of the Alcohol, Drug Abuse, and Mental Health Administration

(ADAMHA), Public Health Service and Department of Health and Human Services. The recipient of numerous awards, he is active in many professional societies, serves on the editorial boards of several journals, and has been a consultant to many groups.

Michael R. Liebowitz, M.D., is currently Assistant Professor of Clinical Psychiatry at the College of Physicians & Surgeons of Columbia University and Director of the Anxiety Disorders Clinic at the New York State Psychiatric Institute. He received his M.D. from Yale University School of Medicine. The author of more than thirty professional publications, in 1977 he received first prize from the New York District Branch of the American Psychiatric Association for resident research project.

James Grier Miller, M.D. (Harvard) is President of the Center for the Study of Democratic Institutions, University of California at Santa Barbara. He has served on the faculties at Harvard, the University of Chicago, the University of Michigan, Johns Hopkins University, and the University of California, and is President Emeritus of the University of Louisville. For more than twenty years Dr. Miller has been editor of the journal *Behavioral Science.* He has written or coauthored eight books and published more than 200 scientific and scholarly articles. He is a fellow or member of numerous scientific and professional societies.

Jessie L. Miller is a graduate of Radcliffe College and has received her M.S. degree from Simmons College in Boston. She has published several previous articles jointly with her husband, with whom she has worked in research and writing for more than 40 years.

Mortimer Ostow, M.D., (New York University) Med. Sc.D (College of Physicians & Surgeons of Columbia University) is the author of *Drugs in Psychoanalysis and Psychotherapy* and the editor of *The Psychodynamic Approach to Drug Therapy.* He also wrote or edited seven other books and more than a hundred scientific papers. He was graduated from the New York Psychoanalytic Institute in 1950 and has practiced psychoanalysis since. He was elected an Honorary Member of the Israel Psychoanalytic Society and in 1979 received the Maimonides Award of Wisconsin. He also serves as the American editor of the *Israel Journal of Psychiatry.*

Eliot H. Rodnick, received his Ph.D. from Yale in 1936 and is Professor Emeritus of Psychology, University of California, Los Angeles. He has published extensively and has served on various governmental advisory committees. He is a past president of the American Orthopsychiatric Association and a recipient of many professional awards.

Gerald J. Sarwer-Foner, M.D. (University of Montreal) is Professor and Chairman of the Department of Psychiatry, University of Ottawa School of Medicine. Previously he was at McGill University and has been visiting professor at many faculties of medicine. He serves on the editorial boards of numerous journals and has written three books, over 130 papers, and many teaching audio and video tapes. He is a fellow of ten professional associations and has held executive positions with many psychiatric organizations.

Myrna M. Weissman Ph.D. (Yale) is a Professor of Psychiatry and Epidemiology at Yale University School of Medicine and Director of the Depression Research Unit, Connecticut Mental Health Center. She has been a governmental consultant and an editorial consultant to several psychiatric journals. She has published more than 150 scientific articles as well as coauthored a book with Dr. Eugene S. Paykel, *The Depressed Woman: A Study of Social Relationships,* and has edited a book with Jerome Myers and Catherine Ross, entitled *Community Surveys.*

Otto Allen Will, Jr., M.D. (Stamford) has held academic appointments at Johns Hopkins University School of Medicine, the University of Maryland School of Medicine, the University of Chicago Department of Psychiatry, and Cornell University, in addition to hospital appointments at Chestnut Lodge, Rockville, Md. and Austen Riggs Center, Stockbridge, Mass. The recipient of several awards, he is now in private practice.

Psychopharmacology and Psychotherapy

CHAPTER 1

The Relevance of Psychiatry in the Psychoses

Roy R. Grinker, Sr.

THE TITLE OF THIS CHAPTER requires the almost impossible task of defining both psychiatry and the psychoses. Psychiatry is a multifaceted field. The research arm attempts to determine the meaning of the term psychiatry and the derivation or etiology of various psychiatric disturbances. One of the best examples of the absence of sufficient information is in the case of the term schizophrenia. Much more research is required before the etiology of this psychiatric disturbance can be determined. Yet the term psychosis does not specify schizophrenia, because there are many kinds of psychoses, such as traumatic, infectious, senile, depressive, and many other processes that initiate difficulties in adapting to reality.

The second problem in defining psychiatry is the problems inherent in proving the efficacy of treatment techniques. The use of different forms of therapeutic intervention together can make it impossible to determine the most effective treatment. For example, the natural evolution of the schizophrenic psychoses may result in improvement or even remission for years, or it may result in a rapid deterioration to a chronic state which could last for years, or even forever. Administration of psychotropic drugs may alter the natural course of the disease and ameliorate the psychosis but not affect thinking and feeling, despite the decrease in psychotic behavior. It is thus difficult to determine the efficacy of one form of treatment.

One can also ask: What are the effects of interpretations based on psychodynamic principles? Are these effective, or are they simply the fragments of the musings of the therapist? In addition, the family and other environmental factors may help or hinder progress toward improvement. The relationships among the many variables involved in treatment result in confusion; when many treatments are used in conjunction with one another, it is impossible to pinpoint the source of therapeutic effectiveness.

In general, psychiatry has divided mental illness into several large categories, such as the psychoses, neuroses, and personality disturbances. The psychoses, which include many conditions that result in unrealistic thinking, feeling, and behavior, are viewed by psychiatrists as either psychotic depressions or schizophrenia. During the early stages of scientific psychiatry, most attention was paid to this form of mental disturbance, especially in state hospitals.

When psychoanalysis began to permeate psychology and psychiatry in the United States, it was the neuroses that demanded almost exclusive attention; to a much lesser extent, psychosomatic disturbances also received attention (Grinker, 1953–1956). Psychosomatic disturbances were classified, according to the theories of Franz Alexander, into types according to the emotional disturbances that precipitated them. For a long time, it was impossible to alter this classification scheme. It was not until the data were reexamined that we found that the psychosomatic disturbances were not due to specific etiological factors but were related either to constitutional or experiential processes which made responses to external or internal precipitating stress important partial aspects of causes. Thus, we now talk about response specificity rather than stimulus specificity (Grinker, 1966).

Psychopathic or personality or character disturbances have attracted little attention except for the so-called borderline syndrome (Grinker, Werble, and Drye, 1968). This syndrome indicates that there are, as well as narcissistic neuroses, specific kinds of psychopathy that apparently have different causes, different effects, and require different forms of treatment.

Nonetheless, appropriate treatment for the amelioration of symptoms has not clarified the basic etiology of psychosis. In fact, there is a movement afoot to stimulate psychiatrists to pay more attention to the psychoses, and a host of literature has accumulated indicating different points of view regarding etiology.

In general, the methods of treatment are rather vague. In addition, there are many different forms of therapeutic intervention. According to Marshall, there are 100 to 140 schools of psychotherapy (1980). Long-term evaluation of the efficacy of treatment methods has been neglected. It is hard to envision with any degree of reliability research which would depend upon only one or two years of follow-up. Nonetheless, prediction in terms of the patient's early status in life may indicate to some degree the prognosis for individual patients to become better, worse, or to remain unchanged.

Hans Strupp and his colleagues have spent much time and energy in studying the effects of therapy. They have concluded that the nonspecific factors, such as attitudes by professionals and even nonprofessionals, are the essential factors conducive to improvement. Their research indicates that it is a particular combination of the values of the patient and of the therapist that will give rise to a particular relationship and often to a positive therapeutic outcome. The positive changes experienced by Strupp's patients, whether treated by a professional or a nonprofessional, are generally attributed to the healing effects of a benign human relationship. Professional therapists, by virtue of their training and clinical experience, are clearly much better equipped to deal with the vagaries and vicissitudes encountered in the interactions with most patients. "However, it does not seem fair to conclude that given a carefully specified protected context, mature and competent individuals even in the absence of professional training can engage appropriate patients in an interpersonal relationship whose outcome is therapeutic" (Strupp and Hadley, 1979).

The many forms of treatment, the milieu and even *natural* evolution of a disease toward a positive or a negative result, drugs, the relationship between patient and therapist, and interpretations on a psychodynamic basis, followed by long-term or cross-sectional evaluation, are important criteria of results. But these seem so simple in contrast with other medical fields that they appeal to nonprofessionals.

The first effort in psychiatry (based on Kraepelin's work) used the medical model exclusively. Kraepelin promulgated a new field of neuropathology which most of his peers attempted to learn. Many were dismayed, however, by the fact that the specific set of changes associated with specific diseases were not universally demonstrable, although the correlation as a direct line between brain pathology and clinical phenomena lasted for decades. The drugs used were mostly sedatives; continuous sleep and other modes of treatment were also used for therapy. With the advent of psychoanalysis and its competition with the biological attitude toward the psychoses, many psychiatrists realized that biological and psychological factors were clearly imbedded in environmental experiences; the result was more than a combination of two factors added together. The psychotic internal transaction is a continuous process with feedback and spiral development through a series of critical stages. It is difficult, then, to link the medical with the behavioral model; it requires the development of a systems or unified theory (Grinker, 1956). These exciting attempts have met success with the efforts of only a few psychiatrists.

Nineteenth-century developments in biology were the essential foundations of and became the necessary conditions for the concept of the unity of science. Although Freud admitted the presence of unknown biological factors, psychoanalysis spread in this country and dominated for a time. We found ourselves enmeshed in a dichotomy, medical versus behavioral, biological versus psychological. But as time went on, it became obvious that we were dealing not with dichotomy but with a unified system. This applied to the theory, diagnosis, and treatment of families, groups, or even communities without a total immersion in individual difficulties.

Thus we are now dealing with the properties of a systems theory (Bertalanffy, 1968) which gives us no handle on etiology, but which enables us to use our therapeutic skills on both the organic and the psychological factors. One can hardly say that we are still in the process of uncovering any particular causes. The parts are held together by control and regulation and include biological, psychological, social, and cultural processes (Grinker, 1979).

One example of such a therapeutic approach is insight therapy. Insight is a vague psychoanalytic concept that simply represents a continuous reinforcement which seeks to alter behavior in the present with internalized feedback; this in turn alters the state of the central nervous system to the extent that external behavior also becomes changed to some degree. This process has inspired attempts to develop a new action language by Ruesch (1969), Schaefer (1973), and Grinker (1956).

It is clear that the simplicity of the therapeutic method, however unsound and ineffective, has caused nonprofessionals to rush into treatment of psychoses while ignoring the problems of causation and evaluation. Moreover, psychiatrists themselves have blurred the boundaries of their field by calling themselves *primary* physicians. We now have another dichotomy, which has been so ably described by Frank (1977), in the subjective history versus the object of examination. This dichotomy can be alleviated by the use of an action language which indicates that a new pattern may feed back to the periphery, regardless of the genetic or experiential constitution and psychological experiences of the patient. Unfortunately, this understanding has given rise to practices such as encounter groups, run by lay people who have no concern with cause, or with evaluation, but are motivated by financial desires. As a result, there have been a series of casualties among patients who have taken part in encounter group treatment (Grinker, 1975).

In my opinion, the notion of a "spectrum" background for schizophrenia recently has been imitated by a "spectrum" for depression. This concept has failed to work because the items within the spectrum have not been clearly defined or analyzed on the basis of adequate empirical data. As a result, of the items on the spectrum for depression—blood dyscrasias, asocial behavior, color blindness, and alcoholism—all except color blindness and blood dyscrasias are subjective characteristics dependent on the cultural milieu.

In an effort to determine whether a depression is endogenous, we have drawn upon our experience that people treated for psychotic depressions with shock treatment, drug treatment, or other milieu experiences do not want to receive further insight therapy regarding the causative factors of their depressions (Grinker, Miller, and Sabshin, 1961). Many patients do not even want to talk about the precipitating factors.

Crittenden (1980) has studied the depressed patient after recovery from the psychosis itself. Her findings indicate that the period between psychotic episodes is characterized by intense insecurity and negative feelings of self in relation to behavior with others. In other words, self-esteem continues to be at a low ebb between depressions. Statistical analysis of her data resulted in the division of the syndrome into subcategories and in a guide for interpretation of the meaning of experiences to the individual's genetic and developmental origins of the manifested disequilibrium. In addition to social and cultural factors, it appears that meaningful others are involved in precipitating the psychosis in individuals with specific premorbid personalities. Demographic indices were also found to be important. If these variables could be better understood and associated with the symptomatology I have described, we could further our comprehension of depression and prove and extend clinical psychiatric research without which meaningful sociological, psychodynamic, and biological correlations are impossible.

In a recent study of depression, we rated a large number of patients in terms of their inner feelings and behaviors on a scale developed from fifteen factors of these combined phenomena or four so-called factor patterns. These factor patterns are as follows:

1. A feeling of dismal hopelessness; a loss of self-esteem; slight guilt feelings; isolated, withdrawn, and apathetic behavior; slow thought and speech; and some cognitive disturbances.
2. Hopelessness; low self-esteem; intense guilt feelings; high anxiety with agitation and clinging demands for attention.
3. A feeling of abandonment; loss of love; and agitated, demanding, hypochondriacal behavior.
4. Gloom, hopelessness, anxiety, and demanding, angry, provocative behavior.

These factor patterns, based on careful analysis of behavior and feelings and on the concerns of inpatients diagnosed as suffering from a state of depression, provide clinical definitions and descriptions (Grinker et al., 1961).

Despite Freud's acceptance that nothing can be done about the biological factors in the etiology of psychoses, psychoanalysis gradually began to ignore the roles of hereditary and constitutional factors significant to the etiology of the psychotic syndrome. It appeared that the discovery of psychotropic drugs (antidepressive, antimanic, and antischizophrenic) would open a relevant approach to the psychoses. However, this would be true only if these drugs pinpointed the brain areas most dominant in the etiological syndrome (Grinker, 1941).

Wolpert (1977) found that patients on lithium had a 72 percent recurrence of their manic-depressive episodes. At the time of recurrence, 41 percent were on lithium and one-third required rehospitalization. Nevertheless, he termed the syndrome an "actual neurosis" carrying a "basic vulnerability." He maintained that failures in treatment are due to neglect of psychological issues. Back we are sent, to a *systems* approach which includes a wide distribution of the relevance of psychiatry and biology.

Indeed, depression is recognized today as a syndrome with various components. However, the presence of depression does not of itself denote a *psychiatric* syndrome, since humans may demonstrate depressed behavior when confronted with frustrations, obstacles, and conflicts; thus, depression can be a component of a host of psychological responses as well as psychiatric syndromes. It was a step forward when depressions were noted to be one side of a dual condition, namely mania, and the syndrome of manic-depression as a psychosis was discovered. There have been innumerable efforts to base the tendency toward depression and the entire syndrome on biological and physiological grounds. However, most of the attempts at classification were based upon characteristics in rating scales, such as the Zung or the Hamilton Scale, but very few efforts were oriented toward classification of depressions into clinical subcategories, the real relevance of psychiatry to a psychotic process.

In an effort to determine the relationship of psychotherapy to psychiatry, it is important to understand what we do with our patients in psychotherapy that gives us insights into etiology and potential results. Even the study of the most serious psychosis of all, schizophrenia, has offered nothing but thousands of books and papers over time that tell us very little new (Arieti, 1974). In fact, one of the great errors in the diagnosis and treatment of schizophrenia is that, if improvement occurs and restitution of competent behavior results, the diagnosis is considered erroneous and the patient is considered not to have been schizophrenic. Indeed, the combination of depression and schizophrenia has evoked a notion of more than one disease, such as schizoaffective psychosis, since many schizophrenics are depressed both at the beginning and during the phase of recovery from schizophrenic disintegration.

Kayton (1973) described this depressive syndrome and indicated that it clearly represents some kind of internal re-evaluation of the status of the patient, regardless of the type of therapy, and that this re-evaluation is an important process with which antidepressive drugs should not be allowed to interfere. He describes several phases in the recovery; these phases indicate an internal dynamic process which is poorly understood and the subject of recent controversy.

The follow-up of schizophrenia after treatment is a long and difficult process. There are many forms of treatment and many forms of recovery. Even chronic schizophrenic patients may, after some decades, suddenly recompensate and become much more healthful. All of this, of course, is dependent upon the state of the environment and familial acceptance of the patient's improved status.

It is difficult to do a follow-up study of schizophrenics. One has to take into account many variables involved in the treatment and in the accidental changes of the patient's social and cultural situation. A follow-up study should continue for at least twenty years. It is clear that there are numerous questions regarding the relationship of psychotherapy and psychoses, especially in the case of schizophrenia. Long-term evaluation could reveal the nature of the underlying defect and prolonged abnormalities.

The many psychiatric approaches included in the array of reported successes in the treatment of schizophrenia, and thereby considered to portray etiology, indicate failures in follow-up studies. Short-term follow-ups suggest improvement, but longer follow-ups and wider samples show a 62 percent rehospitalization rate and more than 50 percent of patients functioning poorly in the community (Harrow et al., 1978). Schizophrenias clearly represent systems or fields with discernible linkages of organic, psychological, and social theories, a combined biopsychosocial system in which psychiatry is only one relevant factor.

To synthesize the theories of psychopathology in all of the psychoses, the neuroses, and the personality or character disturbances is a very difficult problem. For example, the conflict theory of schizophrenia as stated is not tenable as the basic cause of schizophrenia, although it may refer to conflict between the schizophrenic process and reality (Holzman and Grinker, 1974). Systems theory and the language of psychic energy are incompatible. In the schizophrenic there seems to be a deficit in *internal organization* and a disintegration of the inner psychological world, which more or less attempts at restitution. Neuroses and psychoses are not continuous processes, although the schizophrenics have neurotic overlays.

A large question occurs regarding the clear emergence of overt psychiatric illness during adolescence, which is the most frequently disturbed age group. Are adolescence and schizophrenia related to each other, or are the coincidences then simply attributable to chance factors? Is schizophrenia a disorder, or is it like Huntington's chorea, occurring at a particular age because of the time necessary for its inexorable incubation and the maturation of the central nervous system? Is adolescence the pathogenic agent and intrinsic factor which potentiates or triggers schizophrenia, or do the social demands of extrinsic factors during adolescence precipitate schizophrenia in the person who is vulnerable?

Will such a vulnerable person manifest symptoms because social demands have begun to intrude significantly during the adolescent period? Another view of the relationship between adolescence and schizophrenia is that of a catalyst to a biological reaction. The potential for disorganization is characteristic of the person, the social tasks of adolescence place powerful strains on the vulnerable youth, and such a person must draw upon his limited resources to respond to these task requirements. His response thus exposes his deficits, and the strain of the requirements can potentiate disorganization. The consequences of such failure to the adolescent's sense of worth, self-esteem, and pride are great; he has finite burdens to add to his failures already sensed through the preceding years (Harrow and Prossen, 1978).

One of the biggest problems in psychiatry is the intrusion of so many individuals without proper training into the field known as the mental health profession, a term which should be abrogated as quickly as possible. What should be done? First, students in universities should be taught much more comprehensive courses in psychology and biology. Second, practicing professionals, who may be poorly informed need to be reintroduced to the currently acceptable consequences of the psychoses. Third, the media should be briefed, by experienced professionals, not by recently graduated psychologists who spout authoritatively in response to any questions raised by reporters intent on a particular story; and fourth, the public should be better indoctrinated to the meaning of mental health and disease.

These are difficult tasks, but they may constitue our effort since we do not have control over the basic problems linked to illness—poor living conditions, lack of an adequate job, poor food and nutritional deficiency, and proper prenatal and post-natal care. None of these are psychiatric responsibilities, since in these areas of social engineering we are not trained and we are not experienced; all we can do is say which of the social phenomena that exist are highly conducive to mental disturbances.

I would like to end with a quotation from Mora (1966), who has done a great deal to further our knowledge of the history of psychology. He says

> On the one hand the comprehension of the cultural atmosphere of each particular period is enhanced by familiarity with historical researches from humanities in general, from medical history in particular. On the

> other hand the clinical work of the psychiatrist assures the comprehension of the internal struggle of the individual considered in historical reality quite apart from generalization of an impersonal nature. The antithesis between the historical and the humanistic orientation will probably always persist as a fundamental dimension of the history of psychiatry.

But clinical psychiatry cannot stand alone in the search for etiologies and therapies of the psychoses viewed as systems.

References

ARIETI, S. *Interpretation of schizophrenia,* second edition. New York: Basic Books, 1974.

BERTALANFFY, VON L. *General systems theory.* New York: Braziller, 1968.

CRITTENDEN, P. *Adjustment and regulation of self-esteem after a depressive episode.* Presented at the 88th Annual Meeting of the American Psychological Association, Montreal, Canada, Sept. 1-5, 1980.

FRANK, J. D. The two faces of psychiatry. *J. Nerv. Ment. Dis., 164:*3-7, 1977.

GRINKER, R. R., SR. Electroencephalographic studies of corticothalamic relations in schizophrenia. *Amer. J. Psychiat., 98:*385-392, 1941.

———. *Fifty years in psychiatry—A living history.* Springfield, Ill.: Charles C. Thomas, 1979.

———. *Psychiatry in broad perspective.* New York: Behavioral Publications, 1975.

———. *Psychosomatic concepts.* New York: Aronson, 1973.

———. *Psychosomatic research.* New York: Norton, 1953.

———. Specificity of response to stress stimuli. *Arch. Gen. Psychiat., 15:* 624, 1966.

———, editor. *Toward a Unified Theory of Human Behavior.* New York: Basic Books, 1956.

———, MILLER, J., SABSHIN, M., NUNN, R., AND NUNNALLY, J. *The phenomenon of depressions.* New York: Hoeber and Co., 1961.

———, WERBLE, B., AND DRYE, R. *The borderline syndrome.* New York: Basic Books, 1968.

HARROW, M., GRINKER, R. R., SR., SILVERSTEIN, M., AND HOLZMAN, P. Is modern-day schizophrenia outcome still negative? *Amer. J. Psychiat., 135:* 1156-1162, 1978.

HARROW, M., AND PROSSEN. Intermingling and disordered logic as influences on schizophrenic thought disorders. *Arch. Gen. Psychiat., 35:* 1213-1218, 1978.

HOLZMAN, P., AND GRINKER, R. R., SR. Schizophrenia in adolescence. *J. Youth Adoles., 3:* 267-279, 1974.

KAYTON, L. Good outcome in young adult schizophrenics. *Arch. Gen. Psychiat., 29:*103-110, 1973.

KRAEPELIN, E. *Clinical psychiatry.* New York: Macmillan, 1912.

MARSHALL, E. Psychotherapy works, but for whom. *Science, 207,* 1, 1980.

MORA, G. The History of psychiatry: A cult and bibliography. *Int. J. Psychiat., 2:* 335-355, 1966.

RUESCH, J. Action models. In Heseltine, G.F.D. (Ed.), *Excerpta Medica Foundation.* Amsterdam: 1969, p. 126.

SCHAEFER, R. The idea of resistance. *Int. J. Psychoanal., 54:*259-287, 1973.

STRUPP, H. H., AND HADLEY, S. W. Specific vs. nonspecific factors in psychotherapy. *Arch. Gen. Psychiat., 36:*1125-1136, 1979.

Wolpert, E. A. *Manic-depressive illness as an actual neurosis.* New York: International Universities Press, 1977.

CHAPTER 2

Conceptual Issues in Combined Treatment

Gerald L. Klerman

IN CLINICAL PRACTICE, the most common treatment plan for most mental disorders, involves some combination of psychotherapy and medication. This combined treatment program is almost always used in cases of severe mental disorder, such as schizophrenia, mania, depression, anxiety states, and many personality disorders. While relatively little data on the effectiveness of this form of therapeutic intervention is available, surveys have been conducted of clinical practices in public or private mental hospitals, psychiatric units in general hospitals, outpatient clinics, community mental health centers, or the offices of private practitoners. These studies indicate an overwhelming trend toward the increasing use of medication in combination with some form of psychotherapy.

For the most part, this trend has gone unnoticed in the professional and scientific literature. This book is a notable effort to make explicit the extent of this growing clinical practice and to draw attention to the scientific and clinical issues involved in combining drug therapy with psychotherapy.

This chapter attempts to place both the clinical and research issues involved in using therapy and psychotherapy in specific disorders into some broader scientific and policy context. Specifically, I shall address three issues:

1. The extent to which ideological struggles within the mental health field have guided the recent history of drugs and psychotherapy in research and practice.
2. Unresolved scientific issues regarding the best mode for demonstrating safety and efficacy of drug therapy and psychotherapy, whether alone or in combination.
3. Continuing policy debates regarding the extent to which these clinical practices are and should be reimbursed under third-party insurance programs.

Ideological Issues

I define ideology as the complex of attitudes, beliefs, and convictions held by an individual in affiliation with others who share these same beliefs. An ideology is more than a set of intellectual beliefs; it includes other components, social, emotional, and motivational. People who share an ideology feel a sense of kinship with one another, and can be described in terms of a movement or group. Thus we have a psychoanalytic "movement" or a "human potential movement." Surgeons rarely talk about "gastrectomy movements," nor do internists talk about cancer chemotherapy "beliefs." In addition to cognitive and social affiliation components, ideologies also have strong emotional components. People with a commitment toward an ideology feel strongly about their beliefs. These beliefs therefore become matters of personal identification. Challenges to the veracity of the beliefs can elicit strong emotional responses of anger and hurt. The combination of these factors—cognitive, social affiliation, and motivational—often lead to scientific and clinical issues in which ideology is surrounded by polemics and controversy.

Looking back at the late 1950s and 1960s, there was little doubt that the introduction of antipsychotic and related drugs elicited tremendous ideological debate and conflict within the psychiatric and mental health professions. In the United States and Canada, psychotherapeutic orientation based on psychoanalytic and dynamic principles predominated. Within that framework, the possible efficacy of the new drugs challenged both theoretical constructs and actual clinical practice. As a result, the claims for efficacy of chlorpromazine, amitriptyline, or related drugs were challenged as being due not to any pharmacological effect of the drugs upon the central nervous system but rather to other factors—the zeal and enthusiasm of the clinician, a placebo effect, or the sequelae of deprivation in public mental hospitals, where these drugs were observed to have the most dramatic effects. These claims clearly required systematic research to determine the real effect of medication.

It was in partial response to these resistances and criticisms that a small band of psychopharmacologists, led by the NIMH Psychopharmacology Service Center headed by Jonathan O. Cole, M.D., launched a series of double-blind randomized controlled trials. This investigation established beyond any doubt that chlorpromazine and related drugs were not placebos but had demonstrated efficacy. This era has been called by Leo Hollister "the year of overkill"; Hollister believed that the amount of evidence generated was excessive, but it was necessitated by the amount of skepticism and criticism related to the dominant ideological view.

In addition to the challenge to the efficacy of psychotropic medicine was a debate as to whether or not psychotherapy and drugs could be combined in clinical practice. As described by Myrna Weissman, a review of the literature in that era reveals the large number of symposia and papers which dealt with the question as to whether or not the introduction of drug therapy into an ongoing psychotherapeutic treatment program would distort the treatment relationship. Some believed that drugs would disrupt the basis for psychotherapy—transference and countertransference— and the patient's motivation to change to such an extent that it would render impossible the continuation of therapy.

This aspect of drug therapy has been called the negative placebo effect. It engenders the expectation that the mere prescription of a drug and its ingestion by the patient would alter the social psychological situation in a way which would reduce the patient's motivation and render the patient more dependent on the therapist. In addition, many feared the very act of prescribing drugs would cause a regression in the patient/doctor relationship to the medical model. It was thought that drug therapy would bring, on the parts of doctor and patient, expectations that the patient's problems could be magically cured by a biological technique. It was believed that the psychotherapeutic process—and its exploration of conflicts, feelings, and interpersonal issues—would become obsolete and unnecessary. Whereas most of the discussions of placebo effect in that era focused on the positive potential benefits of drug therapy, some discussions did exhibit inversion of the usual placebo effect and the postulation of the negative placebo effect.

It should be noted that when this hypothesis was subjected to testing in controlled clinical trials, particularly in the cases of depression and phobias, there was no demonstration of negative placebo effect. If anything, patients receiving the combination of drugs and psychotherapy were often better able to work in psychotherapy, have a lower drop-out rate from treatment, and were rated as more cooperative and satisfied by both themselves and the psychotherapist.

A small number of psychoanalysts and psychotherapists courageously bucked the dominant tide by advocating the exploration of combined drugs and psychotherapy. Prominent in this group were Gerald Sarwer-Foner (see Chapter 11) and Mortimer Ostow (see Chapter 6) who wrote a series of significant books attempting to explain the actions of drugs in relation to psychotherapy.

In light of the current situation, it is interesting to read these papers published in the late 1950s and early 1960s. Today the question is no longer whether or not drugs can be combined with psychotherapy; the evidence from controlled clinical trials over the past twenty years overwhelmingly attests to the efficacy of drug therapy. If anything, the situation has reversed itself completely. The pressure is no longer upon the psychotherapist to bring forward evidence attesting to the safety and efficacy of the various facets of psychotherapy and to establish the value of psychotherapy itself.

Ideological issues nevertheless persist. Within psychiatry there are still some practitioners who tell their patients that they are opposed to the use of drugs, or who denigrate drug therapy as "merely a crutch," claiming that drugs mask basic problems. Conversely, there are many biologically oriented psychiatrists who tell their patients that they do not believe in psychotherapy, that it is a waste of time and money, or that all that is needed is a prescription for lithium or librium.

For the most part, however, such rigid, exclusionist attitudes have become increasingly uncommon within psychiatry. It must be acknowledged that in fields outside psychiatry, such as psychology, social work, and nursing, many remain skeptical of the value of drug therapy. It seems evident that scientific and theoretical issues in this case, have become intertwined with problems of interprofessional rivalry.

Problems of Evidence and Scientific Issues

It is clear that, before combined treatments are employed, there should be four types of scientific evidence available:

1. Evidence for the efficacy of each treatment.
2. Understanding of the mechanism or actions of the treatments.
3. Verified concepts that bridge the two treatments and provide a reasonable basis for combination.
4. Evidence for the efficacy of the combination.

With respect to drug treatments, there is extensive evidence available which confirms the efficacy and safety of their administration.

The methodology required to demonstrate that an intervention works is different from the methodology required to demonstrate *how* it works. In recent years, enormous progress has been made in understanding the mechanism of how drugs operate, particularly through the development and testing of the hypotheses related to the amine neurotransmitters (Schildkraut, 1978). The early optimism attendant to formulation of these hypotheses has not been fulfilled, however, and considerable doubt and controversy persist.

As a result of the experiments with drug therapy, it is now generally accepted that the most rigorous evidence of safety and efficacy is derived through randomized, controlled clinical trials. This method has been increasingly applied to studies of both psychotherapy and psychotropic medication. From the point of view of experimental design in research studies, studies evaluating the combination of drugs and psychotherapy can be conceptualized as similar to the study of two drugs or drug combinations; the ideal design is a 2 x 2 factorial design in which there are four groups:

Group 1 Drug alone
Group 2 Psychotherapy alone
Group 3 Drugs and psychotherapy combined
Group 4 Control group

While the ethics and feasibility of using a control group may limit its practical use, this design is highly desirable from the scientific point of view, since it may demonstrate the true safety and efficacy of the treatments when various forms of control groups have been used.

There are critics of the value of randomized, controlled trials involving psychotherapy. They claim that psychotherapy cannot be measured because it is not a specific technology; its main ingredients are the warmth, empathy, and understanding of the psychotherapist and the expectational set of the patient. This is the viewpoint most clearly articulated by Jerome Frank.

Critics also maintain that it is impossible to ensure uniformity or quality control because of the difficulty in measuring whether one type of psychotherapy offered by one psychotherapist is equivalent to that offered by another. If one ingests 100 milligrams of Thorazine in Detroit, one can be reasonably certain that it is the same chemical composition as 100 milligrams of Thorazine in San Francisco, Moscow, or Naples. Can the same be said for behavioral psychotherapy, for Freudian psychoanalysis, or for interpersonal psychotherapy?

Finally, those who claim that the results of psychotherapy cannot be quantified also assert that the usual outcome measures used in controlled clinical trials are unsuitable for testing the claims of psychotherapy. Drug trials employ outcome measures which rely greatly on manifest symptomatology and social behavior, whereas the claims for psychotherapy are that it influences more subtle aspects of psychopathology, such as intrapsychic conflict, interpersonal relations, self-esteem, personal satisfaction, and personality functioning, including ego defenses.

Policy Issues

Scientific and ideological issues within the profession are often merged with major unresolved policy issues involving the relationships between the mental health professions and the larger health field, particularly with respect to the financing of health care. It must be acknowledged that, since the mid 1960s, there has been widespread discriminatory opposition to the financing of mental health services, particularly psychotherapy, embodied in the federal reimbursement programs, Medicare and Medicaid, and also in the private programs through Blue Cross-Blue Shield and other insurance companies. The continued existence of these discriminatory practices is usually revealed through higher co-payment requirements, limitations on total benefits, and restrictions on the type of practitioners or on types of settings reimbursable. This situation has produced an ongoing debate within the field and a sense of frustration and, at times, acrimony.

The extent of this problem was noted in the report of the President's Commission on Mental Health (PCMH). In its final report the commission recommended a number of ways in which federal programs could eliminate some of these discriminatory practices. Nevertheless, my experience in Washington reaffirms the existence of strong resistance among policy makers, particularly within the reimbursement fields, whether in the federal government's Health Care Financing Administration (HCFA), in the private insurance decision-making group, or in Congress, notably in the Senate Finance Committee and other related groups. In discussions about removing these discriminatory barriers, two objections are raised: First, critics claim there will be an unlimited demand for services, particularly ambulatory psychotherapy services which will "break the bank." In part, this concern is based upon extrapolations from the rate of growth of insurance programs such as the Federal Employees' Program in Washington or the United Automobile Program in Michigan. In another part, it is based upon a fantasized explosion of demand for ambulatory psychotherapy services. Moreover, critics say that an increase in the number of practitioners contributes to an increase in demand. Contrary to the usual expectations of classic economic theory, there is no fixed demand for mental health services. It may not even be true that there is a fixed demand for health services. But the level of demand has grown dramatically in recent decades, and this growth is in part due to the rising expectations of the public as to the quality and nature of life. "Life, liberty, and the pursuit of happiness" were promised to all Americans by the Declaration of Independence, but the public has now come to regard this promise as ensuring the absence of anxiety, guilt, and insomnia. Furthermore, as the number of practitioners in any health field—whether it be the surgeons, radiologists, internists, or psychotherapists—increases in the community, they seem to generate increased demand. Decision makers in the insurance area, whether in Congress or in the administration, are frightened at the proliferation of nonmedical professionals and of nonprofessionals claiming expertise in psychotherapy and demanding inclusion in reimbursement programs. A part of the response to this has been a push by psychologists and social workers for state certification, licensing, and other efforts to restrict the number of practitioners. Establishing various forms of credentials is one way to meet the criticism.

Second, those who are convinced of the need for discriminatory barriers point to the lack of evidence for safety, efficacy, and cost effectiveness of psychotherapeutic intervention. Decision makers of reimbursement policies have become increasingly concerned with escalating costs and have turned to the criteria of safety, efficacy, and efficiency as one means of reducing cost escalation. The mental health field in general and the psychotherapy field in particular, are most vulnerable to this charge because of the apparently limited body of evidence for the efficacy of psychotherapy, whether used alone or in combination with drug therapy.

In recent years, this has been an ongoing debate in a number of professional newsletters and journals. The discussions were prompted by two developments in Washington. First, the Senate Finance Committee has begun considering amendments to the Social Security Act, that finances Medicare and Medicaid, which would limit reimbursement at some proposed future date to only those mental health services that have demonstrated safety and efficacy as established by randomized, controlled trials. Second, within the Executive Branch, the Health Care Finance Administration has begun asking the Public Health Service to review the evidence for efficacy of various kinds of treatments such as aversive therapy for alcoholism using emetine, surgical treatment for transsexuals, and the orthomolecular treatment of schizophrenia with vitamins.

Conclusion

It is my view that the same procedures that are used today to evaluate aversive therapy for alcoholism will be used in the future to assess family therapy for schizophrenia or behavior therapy for phobias. The shadow of the future is upon us; the policy now emerging that reimbursement for all health procedures, be they psychotherapeutic, radiological, preventative, or other, will require evidence of efficacy. The burden of providing scientifically sound evidence as to the efficacy, safety, and efficiency of our treatments will rest with the professionals.

CHAPTER 3

Applications of Living Systems Theory to Conjoint Therapy

James Grier Miller and
Jessie L. Miller

IN A DELIGHTFUL BOOK which is full of fun, *The Official Rules* by Paul Dickson (1978), there are several hundred "rules," "principles," and "laws" such as the many versions of Murphy's Law, the Peter Principle, and many others less familiar. Examples of these are Woody Allen's Law: "The lion and the lamb shall lie down together, but the lamb won't get much sleep"; J. Paul Getty's Reminder: "The meek shall inherit the earth, but not the mineral rights"; and Nixon's Law: "If two wrongs don't make a right, try three."

Two other sayings, both referring to academia, are directly applicable to principles of general living systems theory. One is a statement which is likely to infuriate department chairmen in universities everywhere: "It is fortunate that the good Lord created the universe exactly divided according to the traditional academic disciplines." The other is: "Every academic discipline speaks its own language and there is no Rosetta stone."

The first statement is manifestly untrue. Research that crosses traditional disciplinary lines is increasingly common. The field of psychopharmacology is an obvious example; bioengineering, which combines engineering and medicine, is another. The problems that arise in complex societies are also rarely confined to a single academic field. Whether the issue is drug abuse, alcoholism, the energy shortage, environmental pollution, the impact of radioactivity, or urban blight, the skills of experts in a variety of fields are needed to handle it effectively. Some combination of lawyers, politicians, economists, biologists, physicists, engineers, sociologists, psychiatrists, or other specialists must be called upon because all of these specialties are relevant.

The second statement is, unfortunately, too often true. Communication is difficult among specialists in different fields, not only because each is usually unfamiliar with the subject matter of all the others, but because specialists' languages and conceptual systems differ. Consequently, ideas and phenomena common to multiple specialties are often difficult to identify.

There can and should be a common conceptual system to bridge the gaps that isolate the specialties and subspecialties in science. An integrated systems theory, such as Grinker and his Chicago group began to consider nearly thirty years ago, would be a means of unifying the biological and social approaches to the study of living things. (Grinker, 1956; Grinker and Sahs, 1966). Development of such a general theory concerned with all the phenomena of life is a desirable goal.

From the point of view of psychiatric practice, it appears impossible to evaluate the validity of diagnosis or therapy unless there is a generally accepted conceptual system. As Chief Psychologist of the Veteran's Administration in 1946, I was asked by Dr. Daniel Blain, then the Chief of Neuropsychiatry, and General Omar Bradley, then the Administrator, to evaluate the validity of the diagnoses being made by the rating psychiatrists in the regional offices who were making psychiatric diagnoses of veterans and rating them on the percentage of their disabilities from zero to 100 percent. Since every 10 percent increase in disability at that time represented more than $30 per month, the disability percentage was a significant factor in determining the future income of the patients being rated.

We selected ten regional offices at random and asked the chief medical officer of each to identify the two best rating psychiatrists in his office. Each of these was requested to provide write-ups of his two best cases; each of these twenty psychiatrists then rated all forty cases without identification of their sources. We found no correlation among the psychiatrists in either their diagnostic ratings or their determinations of the percentage of disability ratings. These finding were not published.

A few years later, I was involved in efforts, sponsored by the Medical Division of the Rockefeller Foundation, to make comparative evaluations of different approaches to psychotherapy. At that time, psychotherapists of different schools were claiming approximately 70 to 80 percent effectiveness for several quite different therapeutic systems. None of the reported research supporting these claims, however, was adequately controlled or scientifically convincing.

The results of this study made me feel insecure about psychiatric diagnosis and therapy and, most importantly, about the conceptual system underlying psychiatric practice. This became a critical influence which led me to spend thirty years working toward the development of a general theory of living systems, first with my associates at the University of Chicago and then at the Mental Health Research Institute of the University of Michigan, where in twelve years the group grew from three members to about 100, representing nearly twenty different academic disciplines.

General Living Systems Theory

Our group spent the equivalent of several lifetimes in an effort to develop a conceptual system applicable to biological and social systems of all sorts (Miller, 1978). Certainly the present conceptualization is not the ultimate theory, but there has been progress. Scientists and scholars should continue to work toward a better and more accurate integrative theory. Perhaps our work will begin a tradition that will bridge the islands of the specialties.

One problem with some systems theories has been a lack of the specificity necessary for successful application. Our group has tried, and will continue trying, to make specific statements, to formulate testable hypotheses, and, if possible, to present quantitative data to support our theory.

General living systems theory asserts that a hierarchy of living systems (see Figure 3-1) began to evolve about 3.5 billion years ago with the appearance of cells, the first and smallest living systems. About 500 million years ago, the cell had increased in size and complexity to the point that multicellular systems developed. There was, after that, a period of time—a relatively brief period in evolutionary history—during

LEVEL	APPROXIMATE NUMBER OF YEARS SINCE PERIOD OF ORIGIN	APPROXIMATE MEDIAN DIAMETER SIZE (IN METERS)
Cell	3×10^9	10^{-6}
Organ	$5 \times 10^{8+?}$	10^{-3}
Organism	5×10^8	10^{-2}
Group	5×10^8 ?	10^{-1}
Organization	1.1×10^4	10^2
Society	7×10^3	10^6
Supranational System	4.5×10^3	5×10^6

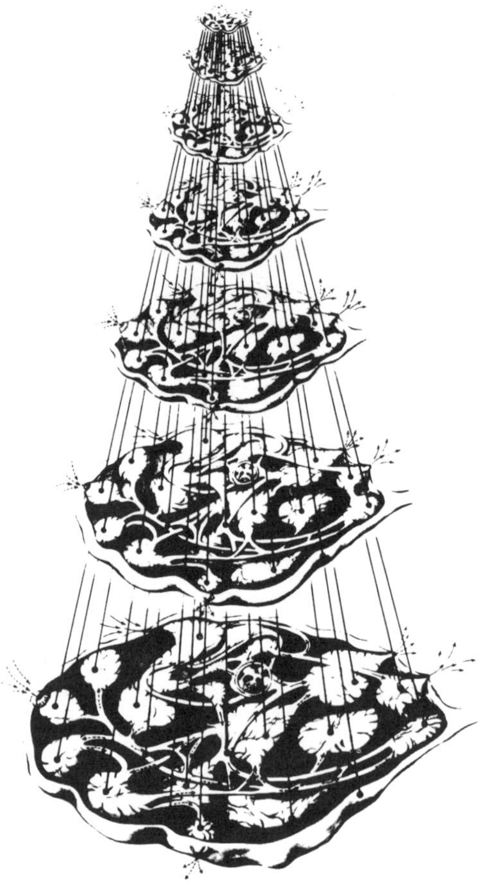

Figure 3–1. The shred-out of cells into a total of seven levels of living systems.

which organ-like organisms similar to existing mesozoans, but able to live independently, existed. Shortly after that, the third level of living systems, the organism, composed of organs, appeared. The fourth level, the group, began when sexual species evolved; a mating dyad was probably the first group. Families, social groups, work groups, and other face-to-face groups followed.

About 10,000 years ago, the fifth level of living systems, the organization, evolved when the number of people living or working together became too large to operate on a face-to-face basis. Organizations are typically composed of several groups which are separated into echelons. Cities of 5,000 to 10,000 people had arisen in the Nile Valley and Mesopotamia by 3100 BC. Copper mines were operated on the Sinai Peninsula under King Seneferu about 3800 BC. Systems of this sort appear too complex to have operated without multiple echelons of authority or decision making and must, therefore, have been primitive organizations.

About 5,000 years ago city-states like Athens and Sparta appeared. These systems exercised control over the territory surrounding them. Such systems gradually evolved into societies or nations, the sixth level of living systems.

Alliances in which societies cooperated toward common goals, usually warlike, were probably the first supranational systems, which constitute the seventh level of living systems. The ancient city of Ur of the Chaldees was probably the first capital of an empire, the Sumerian Empire, which was in existence in the twenty-fifth century BC. The modern form of supranational system includes the United Nations, the Warsaw Pact, and other international bodies in each of which several nations associate with some degree of centralized decision making granted to their assemblies or councils.

The primary components that make up systems at each level are systems at the level below; the lowest level, the cell, has components of nonliving molecules and organelles. Thus organs are composed of cells grouped into tissues; organisms are composed of organs; groups are composed of organisms; and so on. As a result, all living systems have certain common requirements. In order to remain alive, all need to ingest certain materials, such as food and water, to eliminate wastes, to protect themselves from excessive and harmful inputs, to distribute inputs among components, to integrate their components by exchange of information among them, and to carry out a number of other essential life processes.

Each of these essential processes is carried out by specific structures consisting of one or more components of the system. The structures and processes for each essential life process constitute a *subsystem*. We have identified nineteen essential processes for which all living systems must have subsystem structures or must be symbiotic with or parasitic upon another system.

Living systems can be defined as bounded regions in space-time whose subsystems process matter, energy, and information of various sorts. Since matter and energy have related metabolisms in living systems, we combine the two terms for brevity into matter-energy. A subsystem is a matter-energy processing subsystem or an information processing subsystem, depending upon the functions it carries out in its suprasystem, the system of which it is a part.

The matter-energy processing subsystems are concerned with inputs, internal processing, and outputs of matter-energy. The information processing subsystems bring in information from the environment or suprasystem, control and integrate the functions of all subsystems, and send signals out to the environment and suprasystem.

The nineteen subsystems of living systems are listed in Table 3-1. Two of these, the reproducer and the boundary, process both matter-energy and information. The *reproducer* deals with the information in the template, genes, or charter that establishes the structure and basic processes of the next generation. These instructions are incorporated in matter-energy. If a human embryo is to develop into a complete person, the genetic information and appropriate matter-energy must interact. Unlike the other subsystems, the reproducer is not necessary for continuation of each individual system but only for the species or type of system.

The *boundary* acts as a filter for both matter-energy and information. It keeps out unwanted or harmful inputs, permits some inputs to enter, and allows some outputs to pass out of the system into the environment. All living systems are open systems, since the essential processes of life require that they input and output both matter-energy and information. The boundary also protects the system from damage from the environment.

Nine subsystems process matter-energy. The *ingestor* brings matter-energy into the system. The *distributor* takes it to all parts of the system. The *converter* changes the raw materials that enter the system into forms that can be used within the system. The *producer* combines the converted substances to form products that are either required by the system or needed to repair the system itself. Examples are the synthesis of proteins from amino acids, resulting from the conversion of animal protein, and the production of furniture by a factory which converts boards into appropriate shapes. *Matter-energy storage* retains materials in the system for later use or for later extrusion over the boundary. The *extruder* puts out wastes or products from the system. (Whether something is a waste or a product depends upon its use in the environment or suprasystem.) The *motor* moves the whole system or parts of the system in relation to the environment. The *supporter* is the skeleton that maintains relationships

TABLE 3–1

THE 19 CRITICAL SUBSYSTEMS

Subsystems Which Process Both Matter-Energy and Information

Reproducer

Boundary

Subsystems Which Process Matter-Energy	Subsystems Which Process Information
Ingestor	Input Transducer
	Internal Transducer
Distributor	Channel and net
Converter	Decoder
Producer	Associator
Matter-energy storage	Memory
	Decider
	Encoder
Extruder }	
	Output Transducer
Motor }	
Supporter	

among components and holds the whole system in a suitable position in its environment. This engineering process is fundamental even at the cellular level, where the cytoskeleton supports and separates components.

There is a rough similarity between the metabolism of matter-energy and the metabolism of information. The first has been studied in biology for 500 years. Traditionally basic research for medicine, veterinary science, the plant sciences, and agriculture has been concerned with the metabolism of matter-energy. The second metabolism, information processing, has had the attention of social science for perhaps seventy-five years and of biologists for little more than twenty-five years. It is now recognized by biologists and social scientists alike as being of great importance in the understanding of total systems. Most of the specialties of medicine deal primarily with matter-energy processing. This is true of surgery, internal medicine, and pediatrics, for example. Four medical specialties, however, are concerned primarily with information processing. These are genetics, which studies information carried in the genes; endocrinology, which is concerned with information processing by hormones; neurology, which specializes in information processing over neurons; and psychiatry, which deals not only with the genetic, endocrinological, and neurological phenomena related to mental disease, but also with the social phenomena of interpersonal information processing.

Eight subsystems process information. The *input transducer* brings information into the system from the outside and alters the marker, changing it into a form in which it can be transmitted within the system. (A transduction is a change in the matter-energy or "marker" on which the information is carried, such as takes place in a radio when the information carried on electromagnetic waves is transferred to sound waves.) In cells, organs, and organisms, sensory components are input transducers. The olfactory cells in the nose, for example, transduce information from odoriferous molecules propagated through the air to bioelectric pulses that can be transmitted over neural channels. The input transducer is analogous to the ingestor, which brings matter-energy into living systems.

The *internal transducer* transduces information that originates within components of a system from the marker that has carried it inside the component to a marker that can carry it over information channels to other components of the system. Examples of such information are pain signals originating in internal organs and transmitted to the central nervous system in organisms. There is no parallel to the input transducer in matter-energy processing.

The *channel and net* subsystem transmits information to all parts of the system, just as the distributor carries matter-energy. In organisms, this subsystem includes the neural network of the nervous system and the vascular channels that carry hormonal information.

The *decoder* changes information from one code or language to another. Codes are repertoires of information patterns that have the same significance to a sender and a receiver. The languages spoken in human societies are codes, as are the patterns of pulses over organisms' nerves. When auditory input is transduced from sound waves to neural signals, decoding also takes place so that the patterns of pulses retain the significance of the spoken words. The codes used within many systems are different from those in the environment and, in such systems, the decoder changes from the "public" language of the environment to the "private" language used within the system. Recoding may be necessary within systems when the code used in a component differs from the code in which the signal reaches that component. Recoding from neural signals to chemical signals occurs in organisms when a neural signal brings about secretion of a hormone. Recoding occurs in neural transmission when a bioelectric pulse brings about secretion of transmitter substance at a synapse which, in turn, elicits the complex events that lead to a pulse on the postsynaptic neuron.

The *associator* performs the first part of the learning process by combining items or bits of information into patterns of information. Every theory of learning, whether conditioned response theory, stimulus-response theory, stochastic theory, or one of several others, assumes that learning takes place when bonds of some sort are formed between items of information so that one elicits the other with a probability greater than 0 but less than 1. This process is analogous to that of the producer subsystem that combines matter-energy into various forms.

Memory is the second part of the learning process; it is storage of information in the system, analogous to matter-energy storage.

The *decider* is the central subsystem. "To decide" comes from the Latin "to cut." The process in living systems cuts down the number of options, alternatives, or statistical degrees of freedom. The decider receives information through the channel and net about the environment from the input transducer and about all of the nineteen subsystems from the internal transducer. It also may receive information from the past that has been stored in the memory. On the basis of all this information, decoded properly for the decider, this subsystem selects one or more alternatives and eliminates the rest. Directives or command signals are then transmitted to some or all subsystems, changing their processes to bring the system into a state to implement the decision. Such signals may be designed to maintain the steady state of the total system, to move to a new steady state, or in some way to change the relationship of the system to its suprasystem or environment.

The *encoder* changes the code in which information is transmitted from the private code used within a system to the public code of the environment. When a family group does not speak the language of the community in which it lives, someone must translate any message the family wants to send outside the group into the language of the community. That person is an encoder component for the group.

Finally, the *output transducer* transduces information to be output from a marker which is capable of carrying it within the system to one that can be transmitted over environmental channels. The larynx and various muscular motor components which produce facial expressions, gestures, and other bodily movements do this in organisms.

We believe that it is possible to find these nineteen subsystems at all seven levels of living systems, although all types of systems may not have all structures and processes. Plant organisms, for example, lack associator and memory subsystems. Only some plants, such as sensitive plants, transduce information inputs; none has encoder or output transducer subsystems. In most living systems it is possible to determine specifically what structures carry out each of the processes. Those that cannot as yet be identified are chiefly concerned with the memory and learning processes at the levels of the cell, organ, and organism, where the structures are not yet known. Intensive research is going on concerning these particular phenomena, so that within a few years the gaps in our knowledge will very likely be filled.

By means of adjustment processes among subsystems and components of living systems, internal homeostatic equilibria and external equilibria with the environment are maintained. Complex feedback loops connect subsystems and components and serve to guide the system in its environmental relationships.

This has been a brief, and necessarily incomplete, outline of general living systems theory. How can a conceptualization of this sort be used in studying biological and social systems?

Living Systems Theory and Conjoint Therapy

In order to study, understand, and, if necessary, correct disequilibria in a system at any level, the first need is to discover what components are responsible for each of the nineteen subsystem processes. Is the system dependent upon some other system for one or more of these processes? In some systems a single component is the entire structure of a subsystem. In others, multiple components carry out the process. Components of a particular subsystem may or may not be contiguous, and a single component is, in many systems, part of more than one subsystem. The extruder subsystem in human organisms, for example, has many components in different parts of the body. These components include the kidneys, ureters, urethra, sweat glands, rectum, anus, lungs, breathing passages, and breasts.

Harvey's discovery of the circulation of the blood identified the components responsible for the distributor subsystem process in organisms. They are dispersed throughout the entire body, not localized to one component, as many organs are. Following this discovery, physicians came into agreement as to what are the organs that make up the human organism. That agreement among physicians throughout the world led to the modern age of medicine.

At all levels of living systems, the diagnostic strategy of general living systems theory involves the following steps:

1. Identify each of the nineteen subsystems in the system under consideration.
2. Identify a number of variables which are worthy of being measured in each of the subsystems.
3. Find meters, measuring sticks, or indicators with which to make quantitative readings of these variables over time.
4. After making such measurements, determine what the normal steady-state range is for each of the variables and how they interrelate.
5. Make a systematic examination of each of the subsystems, as, for instance, a physician does in a physical examination, to discover which variables are within normal ranges and which are abnormal.
6. Examine all the abnormal variables together in order to identify a syndrome of pathology which these abnormalities may reveal.

After diagnosis has established that pathology of some sort exists in the system, the physician or social scientist may undertake to change the impaired structure in some way or to correct the faulty process.

Conjoint therapy—simultaneous treatment of a patient with drugs and psychotherapy—has always been hampered by the difficulties of conceptualizing the two kinds of therapy in a single, integrated approach. Basically it has fallen afoul of the ancient mind-matter dilemma which still plagues modern psychiatry. Psychiatry has long been segregated from the other medical specialties because this classical distinction has separated mental disease from physical disease, the biological study of human beings from the frequently subjective, psychosocial study of human beings. General living systems theory provides a resolution for this unhealthy situation. It maintains that the proper dichotomy is not between mind and matter but between information processing and matter-energy processing. Either process can affect the other in numerous ways. It is not correct, as has often been assumed, that drugs can affect only biogenic illnesses and that psychotherapy can affect only psychogenic illnesses. Drugs can affect both and so can psychotherapy.

Diagnosis of living systems at any level, according to general living systems theory, should, when possible, identify the structure that carries out each of the life processes. After that is done, a second principle of diagnosis is to trace the routes of all separate sorts of matter-energy and information transmissions, including feedbacks, from inputs to outputs of systems and subsystems. The matter-energy flows include transmissions of drugs, minerals, water, nutrients, and, in higher level systems, persons (who bear information as well as matter-energy). Information transmissions include chemical, electrical, and symbolic transmissions of communications within and among systems, as well as, in higher level systems, of money (which is a special class of information transmission).

A third principle of diagnosis is to base it on the existence of nineteen critical subsystems and to measure whether the variables of each and of the system as a whole are within normal steady-state ranges. One should also determine whether controlling feedbacks are maintaining adjustment processes in healthy states.

Linton and Estock (1977) have applied general systems theory to therapy for anxiety phobic depersonalization. This syndrome begins with an acute attack of anxiety, followed by a withdrawal of the patient, which creates sensory isolation, and is followed by a feeling of depersonalization; the patient then feels he is outside his body, watching himself. Treatment may begin with drugs to reduce anxiety, but drugs also reduce information inputs and decrease the stress response. This, however, may resolve the crisis and follow-up psychotherapy is ordinarily indicated. Drugs can block anxiety signals in a crisis, but psychotherapy may be needed later to decrease the resultant information underload. This is a general living systems theory analysis of the rationale of therapy for this particular syndrome. Diagnosis oriented to our particular approach, directed toward discovering what variables of which of the nineteen critical subsystems are out of normal range or what specific feedbacks or adjustment processes are not operating correctly, can aid in the choice of a type of intervention—drugs, psychotherapy, alteration in the patients' suprasystem or environment, or a combination of such treatments.

The maxim of general living systems theory, that similar pathologies exist and similar strategies for achieving desirable change can be applied at the levels of both biological and social systems, can clarify the strategy of conjoint therapy.

At the level of the cell, addictive drugs like heroin, which are material inputs to cells, create abnormalities in internal cellular information processes by altering enzymatic controls (decider processes). Behavioral changes in the total organism result. Also, excess inputs to human cells of hormonal molecules, bearing chemically coded information, can alter rates of enzymatic processes which affect energy use in the cells and may produce toxic psychoses. Inputs of maladaptive genetic information may create various sorts of illnesses in matter-energy metabolism as well as in information metabolism; examples are phenylketonuria, Down's syndrome, and possibly schizophrenia.

At the level of the organ, abnormal information transmissions, such as inadequate secretion of vasopressin by the posterior pituitary, can produce polyuria; vitamin B-6 deficiency can produce neuritis as well as the psychotic manifestations of severe pellagra. A combination of drug therapy and psychotherapy may be indicated in such illnesses.

At the level of the organism, anxiety is a signal that a steady state has been or threatens to be seriously disturbed. In the presence of an unfilled need or excess stress or threat, the anxiety probably signals the relative strength of the stress or threat, on the one hand, and the adjustment processes available to counter it on the other hand. Anxiety can be a pathological signal in patients with free-floating anxiety. In such persons it inaccurately represents the ratio of stress and threat to available adjustments, so it may be aided by antianxiety drugs. However, anxiety, like pain, is often a useful and accurate signal in normal people and consequently should not be blocked by drugs during psychodiagnosis and psychotherapy.

At the level of the group, drugs may be useful in dealing with anxiety or with physical or psychiatric disorders in one or more family members; but psychotherapy dealing with the abnormalities of information processing and pathological group processes, including pathologies of monetary information flows or family economic problems, are often more important. Certainly the two can be used jointly.

Families continually make adjustments, with the guidance of multiple feedbacks. Some feedbacks are internal, that is, among the subsystems and components of the system itself. Others are external, feeding back into the system from the outside environment. Family members respond to reactions of other members to their own behavior. Depending upon their own dynamics and the dynamics of the total family system, they either change or continue their previous behavior. Such responsiveness in some families can be exceedingly acute. Minimal signs may be correctly interpreted, even when the responding member may not be entirely aware of his own feelings. Such sensitivity can produce harmony in the family if the members' adjustments to signals are negative feedbacks that serve to reduce interpersonal strains. If they are positive feedbacks that serve to increase them, the sensitivity can be destructive.

The importance of feedback in maintaining steady states in families was emphasized by Jackson (1957). His clinical observations led him to view family interactions as information flows with corrective feedback. For example, in one family a boy won a popularity contest, but he found that this displeased his mother. The son then used various adjustment processes in attempts to restore her favor, including efforts to keep from being so popular. Psychotherapy received by one member of a family can change his interactions with the others, thus altering interpersonal steady states of the whole family.

Positive feedbacks can occur in neighborhoods in which there are racial tensions, extreme poverty, or widespread unemployment.

Finally, at the level of the organization, it is clear that inadequate food in a community or insufficient food, drugs, and other supplies in a hospital are lacks of matter-energy inputs that can create pathologies, as can some excesses in matter-energy inputs, like overpopulation. Drugs and other physical measures may correct some such disorders, but the primary disturbances in organizations usually deal with improper routing of information, inadequate or inappropriate feedbacks, distortions, lags, omissions, and errors in communications. These must be diagnosed and corrected by various therapeutic and management methods. Anyone who has spent much time in a hospital knows that its internal health, efficiency, and productivity must be dealt with jointly by therapies or administrative measures that deal with both matter-energy and information processing pathologies.

Conclusions

Conjoint therapy is clearly useful at several levels of living systems that are relevant to psychiatry. The strategy for its use in dealing with matter-energy and information flows needs a unifying conceptual approach, which in the past has not been readily available. Perhaps general living systems theory can contribute such an integration.

It is essential that much more research be undertaken to extend the present limited contributions of systems science to the study of psychiatric problems. This can be done by case studies, by comparing similar processes at various levels of living systems, and also by analysis of the complexity of living systems at all levels, using models and simulations. These methods could be employed by psychiatrists much more extensively to advance our comprehension of the behavior not only of individual human beings but also of lower and higher levels of living systems.

References

DIXON, P. *The official rules.* New York: Delacorte Press, 1978.

GRINKER, R. R., SR., EDITOR. *Toward a unified theory of human behavior: An introduction to general systems theory.* New York: Basic Books, 1956.

——, AND SAHS, A. L. *Neurology,* sixth edition. Springfield, Ill.: Charles C Thomas, 1966.

JACKSON, D. D. The question of family homeostasis. *Psychiat. Quart. Suppl.,* 1957, *31,* 79–90.

LINTON, P. H., AND ESTOCK, R. E. The anxiety phobic depersonalization syndrome: Role of the cognitive-perceptual style. *Dis. Nerv. Syst.,* 1977, *38,* 138.

MILLER, J. G. *Living systems.* New York: McGraw-Hill, 1978.

CHAPTER 4

Pharmacotherapy and Psychotherapy for Ambulatory Depression: Efficacy and Choices

Myrna M. Weissman

THE DIALOGUE BETWEEN the practicing clinician and the researcher has not always been harmonious. On the one hand, the research points to the lack of strong evidence for therapeutic efficacy by maintaining that: (1) properly designed trials have not been conducted; (2) the majority of the completed studies show negative results; (3) the samples are too small or too poorly selected; and (4) only a few treatments have been tested and not even those were sufficiently standardized. As a result, the researcher is reluctant to draw conclusions and calls for more research.

On the other hand, the clinician has had experience with patients who have improved and, on this basis, feels justified in re-using successful treatments. Unlike the researcher in the lab, the clinician is faced with distressed persons and cannot afford to delay acting until the evidence is in. The clinician must act in the face of uncertainty and so uses what he believes will best relieve the patient's suffering. Even the clinician who keeps abreast of the latest research evidence may have difficulty translating it into practice.

The treatment of depression provides a good case example to

demonstrate the tensions between the clinicians and the researcher. Depression is the most common psychiatric disorder in the community and in clinical practice. There are two major treatment choices: drugs and psychotherapy—and a wide variety of psychotherapies can be used alone, in competition, or in combination. These two treatment choices derive from different theoretical realms, require different clinical training, and have different patient acceptance and divergent research underpinnings. There is a plethora of rhetoric concerning which treatment is the most efficacious, and some impressive evidence for efficacy has been accumulating.

As a researcher, I would like to summarize the available research evidence about drugs and psychotherapy for the treatment of depressed outpatients and to translate this evidence into clinical terms which can guide the course of treatment.

Although the overall data may demonstrate that the combination of drugs and psychotherapy is more efficacious than either treatment alone, in fact some patients cannot tolerate the side effects of drugs, while others are unwilling to talk about personal problems. Some clinicians feel that drugs tend to cloud psychotherapeutic issues; others feel that certain patients simply will not benefit from psychotherapy; and still others prefer not to use combined treatment approaches.

Motivation for Testing Psychotherapy

In clinical practice, the most frequent treatment for the ambulatory nonbipolar depressive is a tricyclic antidepressant and some form of psychotherapy. Even though clinicians and patients have consistently testified as to the value of these treatments, the legitimacy of either treatment has come under heavy attack from many sources.

Over the last five years there has been an acceleration in the development of psychotherapies specifically designed for ambulatory depressed patients. Description of the psychotherapies has been improved in procedural manuals that record therapeutic techniques and their sequence during the course of the treatment, and scientific standards have been improved for conducting clinical trials involving psychotherapy, with and without pharmacotherapy. As a result of these efforts, evidence for the efficacy and safety of psychotherapy and pharmacotherapy, each alone and in combination, for the treatment of the ambulatory depressive has become available.

TABLE 4–1 Motivation for Testing Psychotherapy in Depression

Epidemiology:	High prevalence of depression
Economics:	Reimbursement for treatment
Ethics:	Concern about the value and safety of treatments

The majority of the clinical trials of psychotherapy in depression have been carried out among ambulatory depressed patients who are not psychotic and do not have manic episodes. The motivation for clinical trials of psychotherapy, and more specifically on these types of depressions, derives from three sources: their epidemiology, the economics of reimbursement, and the ethics of providing safe and effective patient care (Table 4–1).

Epidemiology of Depression

As noted before, recent epidemiologic studies show that depression is the most common psychiatric disorder in the community, in outpatient general medical practice, in mental health clinics, and in the psychiatrist's office. The nonpsychotic, nonbipolar type of depression has a high prevalence rate, both currently and over a lifetime. The current point prevalence rate has been estimated at about 3 to 4 percent of the adult population, and the lifetime prevalence rate at nearly 20 percent of adults (Weissman and Meyers, 1978). These high rates for nonbipolar depression are in contrast to the rates of bipolar disorder, which are less than 1 percent lifetime risk (Krauthammer and Klerman, 1979).

Clinical trials have emphasized studies of the ambulatory patient because the majority of nonpsychotic, nonbipolar depressives, if treated at all, receive outpatient psychotherapy. Again, this is in contrast to bipolar and psychotic depressions in which hospitalization, medication, and/or ECT are the most widely used treatments, with psychotherapy playing a secondary or adjunctive role.

Economics of Reimbursement

National debates about various forms of private and federal health insurance have provided a fiscal incentive for the scientific testing of psychotherapy in the treatment of all psychiatric disorders. It is hoped that third-party payments for psychotherapy will be increased if evidence for its efficacy is demonstrated in clinical trials. The alternate concern is that third-party payments will be denied unless there is scientific evidence for the value or safety of the psychotherapies.

In fact, the United States Senate Finance Committee led by Chief of Staff Jay Constantine, responding to political pressure, has begun to exert pressure on the profession to provide better proof of the usefulness of the psychotherapies before expanding reimbursement for them (Marshall, 1980A, B). Under consideration over the next ten years are FDA-type trials for psychotherapy, similar to those currently required for the pharmacotherapies, in order to establish the safety and efficacy of the psychotherapies. In the interim, panels of experts would be set up to pass judgment on current practices and to certify useful ones for reimbursement, pending final ruling by clinical trials (Marshall, 1980A, B). Thus, the standards for the testing of pharmacotherapy would be applied similarly to the psychotherapies.

Ethics of Patient Care

Recent court actions have confirmed the patient's right to receive or to refuse treatment. There has also been emphasis on the patient's "right to the right treatment," raising ethical concerns about the treatments that are widely used and accepted as valuable and safe without having been scientifically tested.

Against this background, I would like to describe the psychotherapies which have been designed and tested in clinical trials for the treatment of the ambulatory depressed patient and to present the research evidence for psychotherapy alone and in comparison and in combination with drugs. Before I do so, let us consider what is meant by depression.

Depression as a Clinical Syndrome

Depression, as the clinical syndrome, includes a number of specific symptoms of certain severity and persistence which produce impairment and/or disability and occur in the absence of other symptoms or disorders that might better explain the condition.

Table 4–2 shows the Research Diagnostic Criteria (RDC) for the

TABLE 4-2 Research Diagnostic Criteria (RDC) for a Depressive Syndrome

A. Dysphoric mood which is prominent and relatively persistent.
B. At least five of the following symptoms are required for definitive diagnosis:
   1. Poor appetite or weight loss, or increased appetite or weight gain.
   2. Difficulty sleeping or sleeping too much.
   3. Loss of energy, fatigability, or tiredness.
   4. Psychomotor agitation or retardation.
   5. Loss of interest or pleasure in usual activities, or decrease in sexual drive.
   6. Feelings of self-reproach, or excessive or inappropriate guilt.
   7. Complaints or evidence of diminished ability to think or to concentrate, such as slow thinking or confused thoughts.
   8. Recurrent thoughts of death or suicide, including thoughts of wishing to be dead.
C. Dysphoric features of illness sustained for at least two weeks.
D. Impaired functioning or the seeking of help from someone during the dysphoric period.
E. Absence of the following, whose presence suggest schizophrenia:
   1. Delusions of being controlled or of thought broadcasting, insertion, or withdrawal.
   2. Nonaffective hallucinations of any type throughout the day for several days or intermittently throughout a one-week period.
   3. Auditory hallucinations in which either a voice maintains a running commentary on the subject's behaviors or thoughts as they occur or two or more voices converse with each other.
   4. A span of more than one month during the period of illness during which no prominent depressive symptoms were exhibited but delusions or hallucinations were present.
   5. Preoccupation with a delusion or hallucination to the relative exclusion of other symptoms or concerns.
   6. Definite instances of marked formal thought disorder accompanied by either blunted or inappropriate affect, delusions or hallucinations of any type, or grossly disorganized behavior.
F. Does not meet the criteria for diagnosis of schizophrenia, residual subtype.

[a] Criteria A through F are required for the episode of illness being considered to qualify as a depressive syndrome.

syndrome of major depression (Spitzer, Endicott, and Robins, 1978). Included are dysphoric mood, at least five other symptoms, and persistence of at least two weeks, producing impairment of functioning or necessity of treatment and occurring in the absence of schizophrenia or other disorders that might better explain the symptoms.

Description of the Psychotherapies

Many types of psychotherapies, particularly the psychoanalytically oriented approaches, are widely and appropriately used in the treatment of depression. Unfortunately (as of this writing), only five therapies—cognitive, interpersonal, behavior, marital, and group—have undergone scientific testing in clinical trials among reasonably large, homogeneous samples of depressed patients. Table 4–3 defines these five psychotherapies.

Cognitive Therapy

Cognitive therapy, developed by Beck (1976), is based on the assumption that the affective response in depression is determined by the way an individual perceives experience. As a result of an emergence of maladaptive cognitive themes, the depressed patient tends to regard himself and his future negatively. Correction of negative concepts is expected to alleviate the depressive symptoms. For example, an extremely low self-concept can be treated by presenting a hierarchy of cognitive tasks and demonstrating, through these tasks, the invalidity of the patient's self-reproaches.

TABLE 4–3 Definitions of the Psychotherapies Testing for Depression

Cognitive Therapy: Assumes that the affective response in depression is determined by the way an individual perceives his experience. Correction of negative concepts is expected to alleviate the depressive symptoms.

Interpersonal Psychotherapy (IPT): Assumes that the development of depression occurs in a social and interpersonal context and is determined by the interpersonal relations between the depressed patient and significant other.

Behavioral Approaches: Explains the occurrence of depression in stimulus and response terms. A low rate of positive reinforcement elicits depression; it is predicted by negative reinforcing events in the environment and lack of available positive reinforcements as well as by the individual's behavior.

Marital Therapy: Assumes that the marital relationship affects thoughts, feelings, and behavior and that symptom removal can be achieved by changing the transactional system within the relationship.

Group Therapy: A psychotherapist and a group of patients attempt to effect changes in the emotional states, attitudes, and behaviors of each of the group members.

Interpersonal Psychotherapy (IPT)

Interpersonal psychotherapy assumes that the development of depression occurs in a social and interpersonal context and is determined by the interpersonal relations between the depressed patient and significant others (Klerman, Rounsaville, Chevron, et al., 1979). Depression is seen as having three component processes: symptom formation, social adjustment, and personality. Interpersonal psychotherapy attempts to intervene in the first two processes and does not claim to have an impact on enduring aspects of personality.

The goals are to improve the quality of the patient's social and interpersonal functioning by enhancing the ability to cope with internally and externally induced stresses. This is accomplished by restoring morale and by helping the patient to deal with the personal and social consequences of the disorder. Thus far, techniques have been developed for the management of patients who are depressed with grief and loss, interpersonal deficits, interpersonal role disputes, which are usually marital disputes, and role transitions.

Behavioral Approaches

Behavioral therapy explains the occurrences of depression in stimulus and response terms. A low rate of positive reinforcement elicits certain aspects of the depressive syndrome; it is predicted by negative reinforcing events in the environment and the lack of available positive reinforcements as well as by the individual's behavior (Lewinsohn, Biglan, and Zeiss, 1976).

Several techniques based on behavioral concepts have been developed for depressed patients, such as: social skills therapy, which emphasizes increasing assertiveness, verbal skills, and social adjustment; pleasant events which focus on increasing pleasant and rewarding experiences; and self-control, which emphasizes self-monitoring, self-evaluation, and self-reinforcement in an effort to correct problems in monitoring negative events, in making internal attributions of responsibility, and in excessive self-punishment.

Marital Therapy

Marital therapy attempts to alter the interaction of marital partners. It is based on the assumption that the marital relationship affects thoughts, feelings, and behavior and that symptom removal can be achieved by changing the transactional system within the relationship. Marital therapy can be individual, collaborative, concurrent, conjoint, combined, and group. The theoretical base and a typology of marital types have been well summarized by Gurman and Kniskern (1979).

Group Therapy

In group therapy, a psychotherapist and a group of patients attempt to effect changes in the emotional states, attitudes, and behaviors of each of the group members. Currently, explicit definitions of techniques and descriptions of what occurs within the group format are lacking, although there are efforts to develop cognitive therapy in a group context.

Status of Development of the Five Psychotherapies

Table 4-4 shows the status of the development and testing of the five therapies. Cognitive therapy has been tested in six trials, interpersonal psychotherapy in three trials, behavioral approaches in eight trials, and marital and group therapy in one trial each. Of the five therapies, only cognitive and interpersonal and some of the behavioral techniques have been specifically designed for depressed patients, and only cognitive and interpersonal have available procedural manuals. However, this is a rapidly progressing field; some of the trials noted are still ongoing. Undoubtedly other clinical trials, new therapies, and more procedural manuals are being developed or completed as of this writing.

TABLE 4-4 Development and Testing of Psychotherapies in Depression

	Cognitive	Interpersonal	Behavioral Approaches	Marital	Group
Number of trials with depressed patients	6	3	8	1	1
Designed for depressed patients	Yes	Yes	(Some)	No	No
Procedural manual	Yes	Yes	No	No	No

Evidence for Efficacy

Table 4–5 summarizes the evidence for the efficacy of the five psychotherapies alone, in comparison, and in combination with drugs for the ambulatory depressed patient. [See Weissman (1979) for a more detailed description of these results.]

Psychotherapy Alone

There are nine studies testing the efficacy of psychotherapy in comparison with a low-contact or a no-active-treatment control group (Weissman, 1979). All five treatment approaches are represented. All the studies support the efficacy of psychotherapy alone as compared with a control group. In none of the studies was psychotherapy equal to or worse than a control or no-treatment group; in all of the studies it was shown to be superior.

Psychotherapy in Comparison to Drugs

There are five completed studies in which the efficacy of psychotherapy was compared to that of a tricyclic antidepressant. All five of the psychotherapies are represented (Weissman, 1979). One study found psychotherapy (cognitive therapy) superior to drug use (imipramine) in

TABLE 4–5 Evidence for Efficacy of Psychotherapy and Drug Use in the Treatment of Depression

	NUMBER OF STUDIES
Psychotherapy Alone	
Psychotherapy > control	9
Psychotherapy = control	0
Psychotherapy < control	0
Psychotherapy in Comparison to Drug Use	
Psychotherapy > drugs	1
Psychotherapy = drugs	1
Psychotherapy ? drugs	3
Psychotherapy > drugs in social functioning	
Psychotherapy < drugs in symptom prevention	
Psychotherapy in Combination with Drugs	
Psychotherapy + drugs > psychotherapy > drugs > control	4

attrition and symptom reduction for the acute treatment of depressed patients. One study found drug use and psychotherapy about equal for acute symptom reduction. Three studies found drugs superior to psychotherapy (interpersonal, group, or marital) in the prevention of relapse or symptom reduction, but psychotherapy slightly superior to drugs in the enhancement of social functioning. The psychotherapy effect in one study occurred only in those patients who remained in treatment for eight months without relapsing.

The results of the comparisons of psychotherapy with pharmacotherapy are equivocal for acute treatment. The treatments appear to be equal overall but to have different targets of action. The one study in which cognitive therapy was found to be superior to drug use requires replication before the results can be accepted.

Psychotherapy in Combination with Drugs

There have been four completed studies testing the efficacy of combined psychotherapy (interpersonal, marital, or group) and a tricyclic antidepressant. All four studies showed the superiority of combined treatment over a control group or over either treatment alone (Weissman, 1979). In none of the studies were there negative interactions in combining drugs with psychotherapy. The effects of the two treatments together were additive. Overall, the combination of psychotherapy and a tricyclic was better than either treatment alone or than no regular treatment. The combination provided a broader spectrum of action as each treatment seemed to affect different domains (DiMascio, Weissman, Prusoff, et al., 1979). Psychotherapy seemed to have its effect on social and interpersonal areas and had a slower onset of action. Drugs had their effect on vegetative symptoms of depression, such as sleep and appetite, and had a more rapid onset of action.

Guides to the Choice of Treatments

The evidence thus far is in favor of the combined treatment (drugs and psychotherapy) over either treatment alone for the ambulatory depressive. However, there is considerable variability in the patient's and in the clinician's preferences for treatment. What research evidence can guide the choice of treatment for the ambulatory depressive?

Which Antidepressant?

The selection of which antidepressant, for which patient, and in what sequence, is too broad and complicated a topic to be handled here.

Which Psychotherapy?

We cannot yet state how the psychotherapies compare to one another, nor can we offer guides on the basis of research data about the selection of a particular psychotherapy for the depressed patient. The NIMH-sponsored collaborative study on the psychotherapy of depression will ultimately provide data on the relative efficacy of cognitive and interpersonal psychotherapy.

Pharmacotherapy versus Psychotherapy

The evidence comparing pharmacotherapy to psychotherapy is equivocal and inconclusive. However, the patient who will not accept one treatment should not be denied the other, since the evidence shows that either treatment is better than no treatment. Moreover, there are several findings on the symptoms, social functioning, and diagnostic subtypes of patients from our own data and that of others which can begin to guide the clinician's selection of an effective treatment.

Symptoms and Social Functioning. The research evidence shows that pharmacotherapy is most efficacious on sleep disturbance and appetite loss and that the effects on these symptoms are relatively early in the treatment process (one to four weeks). Therefore, the patient whose depression is mostly manifest in these symptoms should be given an antidepressant (DiMascio, Weissman, Prusoff, et al., 1979).

Alternately, psychotherapy is most efficacious in dealing with suicidal feelings, guilt, loss of interest, and social and interpersonal problems; it is strongly indicated for patients whose depression is mostly manifest in these areas. Psychotherapy has a later onset of action, and the differential effects on social and interpersonal functioning may not be apparent for six months to one year (Weissman, Klerman, Prusoff, et al., 1981).

Diagnostic Subtypes. Recent findings by Prusoff, Weissman, Klerman, et al., 1980) from the New Haven-Boston Collaborative study suggest that the Research Diagnostic Criteria (RDC) subtypes of endogenous and situational depression may be useful guides to treatment selection (Beck, 1976).

Endogenous and situational depressions are defined by the RDC (Spitzer, Endicott, and Robins, 1978) as follows:

I. Endogenous Major Depressive Disorder—from groups A and B a total of at least four symptoms for probable diagnosis, six for definite, with at least one symptom from group A.

Group A: (1) Distinct quality to depressed mood, that is, depressed mood is perceived as distinctly different from the kind of feeling the patient would have or has had following the death of a loved one; (2) lack of reactivity to environmental changes [once depressed the patient does not feel better, even temporarily, when something good happens]; (3) mood is regularly worse in the morning; (4) pervasive loss of interest and/or pleasure.

Group B: (1) Feelings of self-doubt, reproach, or excessive or inappropriate guilt; (2) early-morning awakening or middle of night insomnia; (3) psychomotor retardation or agitation [more than a mere subjective feeling of being slowed down or restless]; (4) poor appetite; (5) weight loss [two pounds a week over several weeks or twenty pounds in a year when not dieting]; (6) loss of interest or pleasure [may not be pervasive] in usual activities or decreased sexual drive.

II. Situational Major Depressive Disorder—illness has developed after an event or in a situation that seems likely to have contributed to the appearance of the episode at that time. In making the judgment, the amount of stress inherent in the event or situation is considered, as are the cumulative effect of such stresses and the closeness of the events to the onset or exacerbation of the depressive episode.

In the New Haven–Boston clinical trial, eighty-one depressed patients were randomized into one of four treatments: combined amitriptyline and interpersonal psychotherapy (IPT), either treatment alone, or a nonscheduled treatment control group (DiMascio, Weissman, Prusoff, et al., 1979; Prusoff, Weissman, Klerman, et al., 1980). Of the eighty-one patients, thirty-one (40 percent) were diagnosed by the psychiatrist at the intake interview as situational only and twenty (27 percent) as endogenous only.

Figure 4–1 shows the end-of-treatment results on overall depressive

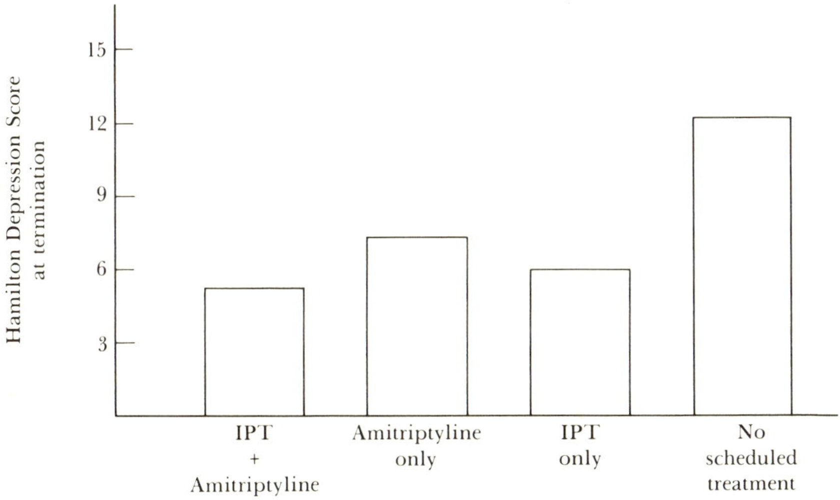

Figure 4–1. Endogenous Depression Only

symptoms, based on the Hamilton Depression Scale, for the depressed patients diagnosed as situational only. These patients responded equally well to all treatments and responded poorly to nonscheduled treatment. However, the combination of drugs and psychotherapy did not seem to offer more than psychotherapy alone.

Figure 4–2 shows the results for endogenous depression. As can be

Figure 4–2. Situational Depression Only

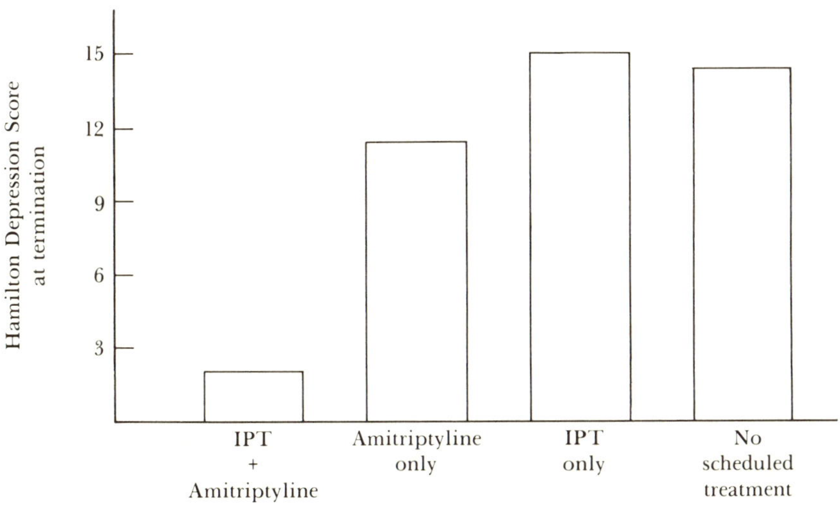

seen, these patients responded poorly to psychotherapy alone, which was not any better than no scheduled treatment. The response was best to the combination of drugs and psychotherapy. The lack of better response to drugs alone may have been due to poor compliance. This study was begun in 1972 before plasma level monitoring of tricyclics was feasible. Future studies will incorporate plasma level tests.

These results are based on small samples and require replication. They suggest that the situational depressions respond best to psychotherapy alone and that the concurrent use of drugs adds little. Treatment of endogenous depression, on the other hand, does not progress well on psychotherapy alone.

Conclusion

Evidence for the efficacy of pharmacotherapy and psychotherapy for the ambulatory, nonbipolar, nonpsychotic depressive is rapidly developing. There is sufficient evidence from small, individually conducted clinical trials to warrant the launching of a multicenter collaborative trial which would test the efficacy of several therapeutic approaches with and without drugs in large samples of this population. Such a study has been designed by the staff at the Clinical Research Branch, National Institute of Mental Health, in consultation with many experts, and it has been approved by peer review. In addition, a number of single-center clinical trials are currently under way (Weissman, 1979). If the rate and direction of progress in this area continue, the next decade will bring clearer answers as to which types of psychotherapies to use with which drugs, and for which depressed patient, and there will be a scientifically supportable rationale for the treatment of the different types of depression. Pending these results, many of the research findings can be translated into clinical care.

ACKNOWLEDGMENT

This research was supported in part by Alcohol, Drug Abuse, and Mental Health Administration grant MH 26466 from the Clinical Research Branch, National Institute of Mental Health, Rockville, Maryland. This work is a summarization of the results from:

Weissman, M. M. The Psychological Treatment of Depression: Evidence for the Efficacy of Psychotherapy Alone, in Comparison with, and in Combination with, Pharmacotherapy. Archives of General Psychiatry, *Volume 36, 1261-1269, 1979.*

Prusoff, B. A., Weissman, M. M., Klerman, G. L., and Rounsaville, B. J. Research Diagnostic Criteria Subtypes of Depression: Their Role as Predictors of Differential Response to Psychotherapy and Drug Treatment. Archives of General Psychiatry, *Volume 37, 796-801, 1980.*

References

BECK A. *Cognitive therapy and the emotional disorders.* New York: International Universities Press, 1976.

DIMASCIO, A., WEISSMAN, M. M., PRUSOFF, B. A., et al. Differential symptom reduction by drugs and psychotherapy in acute depression. *Arch. Gen. Psychiat. 36:*1450–1456, 1979.

GURMAN, A. S., AND KNISKERN, D. P. Research on marital and family therapy: Progress, perspective, and prospect. In Garfield, S. L., and Bergin, A. E. (Eds.), *Handbook of psychotherapy and behavioral change: An empirical analysis,* 2 ed. New York: Wiley, 1979.

KLERMAN, G. L., ROUNSAVILLE, B. J., CHEVRON, E., et al. *Manual for short-term interpersonal psychotherapy (IPT) of depression,* 4th rev. June, 1979. (Unpublished.)

KRAUTHAMMER, C., AND KLERMAN, G. L. The epidemiology of mania. In Shopsin, B. (Ed.), *Manic illness.* New York: Raven Press, 1979; pp. 11–28.

LEWINSOHN, P., BIGLAN, A. AND ZEISS, A. Behavioral treatment of depression. In Davidson, P. (Ed.), *The behavioral management of anxiety, depression and pain.* New York: Brunner/Mazel, 1976, pp. 91–146.

MARSHALL, E. Psychotherapy faces test of worth. *Science, 207:*35–36, 1980.

———. Psychotherapy works, but for whom? *Science, 207:*506–508, 1980.

PRUSOFF, B. A., WEISSMAN, M. M., KLERMAN, G. L., et al. Research diagnostic criteria subtypes of depression: Their role as predictors of differential response to psychotherapy and drug treatments. *Arch. Gen. Psychiat. 37:* 796–801, 1980.

SPITZER, R. L., ENDICOTT, J., AND ROBINS, E. Research diagnostic criteria: Rationale and reliability. *Arch. Gen. Psychiat. 35:*773–782, 1978.

WEISSMAN, M. M. The psychological treatment of depression: Evidence for the efficacy of psychotherapy alone, in comparison with, and in combination with pharmacotherapy. *Arch. Gen. Psychiat. 36:*1261–1269.

——, Klerman, G. L., Prusoff, B. A., et al. Depressed outpatients one year after treatment with drugs and/or interpersonal psychotherapy (IPT). *Arch. Gen. Psychiat. 38:*51–55, 1981.

——, and Myers, J. K. Affective disorders in a United States community: The use of research diagnostic criteria in an epidemiological survey. *Arch. Gen. Psychiat. 35:*1304–1311, 1978.

CHAPTER 5

Psychotherapeutic Treatment of Manic-Depressive Patients on Lithium

Kay R. Jamison and
Frederick K. Goodwin

BIOLOGICAL ASSUMPTIONS AND CLINICAL PRAGMATISM about the etiology of manic-depressive illness long ago determined the dominance of organic therapies in the treatment of bipolar illness. Thus physicians, ancient and modern, have sought cures not by talking and listening but through direct actions of control: mineral baths, bloodletting, herbs, chains, vapors, bromides, opiates, warm waters, cold waters, and physical and chemical restraints.

For quite obvious reasons, psychotherapy has never been an integral nor a comfortable part of the treatment of manic-depressive illness. Clearly, the psychotic disorders, and their empirically derived remedies, long predate psychological treatments, embedding manic-depressive illness—much more than the neurotic disorders—in medicine, both by history and necessity. Unipolar depressions have had an easier alliance with psychotherapy. This is in part because they generally comprise a wider spectrum of psychopathology with a range of milder syndromes with prominent psychological factors. Because depression encompassed a relatively normal spectrum of emotions and feelings, it traditionally has stimulated counsel from priests, physicians, and friends.

How, then, was manic-depressive illness perceived by the pioneers in the field of psychotherapy, the psychoanalysts? Patients suffering from manic-depressive illness did not fare particularly well as potential candidates for pychoanalytic treatment as described by most psychoanalytic writers. Fromm-Reichmann (1949) characterized manic-depressives as lacking in "complexity and subtlety"; Abraham (1968) described them as "impatient, envious, exploitive, and with dominating possessiveness"; and Rado (1928) felt them to be continually involved in a "raging orgy of self-torture." As analytic patients, manic-depressives were generally compared with schizophrenics and found to be lacking in introspection, too dependent and clingy (Fromm-Reichmann, 1949), disconcertingly able to find vulnerable spots in the therapist (Fromm-Reichmann, 1949; Janowsky, 1970), and often able to elicit strong feelings of countertransference in the analyst (Rosenfeld, 1963: English, 1949).

Thus limited enthusiasm for treating manic-depression, prior to the availability of lithium, is easy to understand. One can imagine the frustration encountered in attempting to treat a hypomanic or manic patient psychotherapeutically; it is sufficiently challenging to get or keep such a patient in the office, let alone to engage him in a meaningful therapeutic endeavor. Likewise, any clinician can appreciate the different kind of frustration involved in treating a profoundly depressed patient. The natural history of the illness carries with it an exceedingly high spontaneous remission rate which, no doubt, encouraged therapists to attribute changes to their therapeutic intervention. Conversely, therapists would tend to assume responsibility when a relapse or no change occurred.

Why do we emphasize what the analysts have had to say about manic-depressive illness? If the biological substrate and its treatment are so clear, why journey back so far into the history of science for attitudes and impressions? First, and as always, the psychoanalysts provided a source of clinically descriptive information, all the more important because present medical ethics discourage the psychotherapeutic treatment of unmedicated manic-depressives. Second, the psychoanalytic school has had in the past, and continues in the present to have, a profound effect on clinical thinking about manic-depressive illness. Not only are most psychotherapists stongly influenced by psychoanalytic conceptions of manic-depressive illness, so too are many of those who contribute to the biological and pharmacological literature on the illness.

In the three decades since Cade's discovery (1949), lithium has moved from a position of therapeutic promise to an extensively studied treatment of choice in bipolar affective disorders. Marketing firms and pharmaceutical companies estimate that more than 120,000 Americans currently are taking lithium (G. Graham, M.D., Smith Kline & French Laboratories, personal communication), figures consistent with Jenner and Eastwood's (1978) estimate that 1 person in every 2,000 in the United Kingdom is now receiving lithium.

Now that lithium is well established and patients remain in remission for long enough periods of time to make psychotherapy a viable adjunctive treatment (and for therapists to see the underlying personality-character structure of patients no longer undergoing chaotic mood changes), it is appropriate to re-examine the role of psychotherapy for patients on lithium. Johnson (1980) discusses the lack of studies dealing with the combined use of lithium and psychotherapy in the psychiatric and psychological literature. Yet, as he states, the needs for therapy are varied and considerable; among the more important are: (1) analysis of maladaptive behavior patterns which patients acquire during the illness and which remain unaffected by lithium treatment, yet which may be amenable to psychotherapeutic intervention; (2) the resolution of interpersonal problems following successful lithium therapy; and (3) support for a long-term prophylactic medication regime.

Characteristics of the illness create certain problems which invite psychotherapeutic intervention. It is a chronic, serious, potentially life-threatening illness. Denial is a natural response. The personal, interpersonal, and social sequelae of manic-depressive illness are often severe, and they can create catastrophic reactions in patients experiencing recurrent manic and depressive episodes. Suicide, violence, alcoholism, and hospitalization are but a few of the well-established correlates of the illness. Although biological variables predominate in etiology and in much of the symptomatic presentation, the primary manifestations are behavioral and psychological, with profound changes in perception, attitudes, personality, mood, and cognition. Psychological interventions can be of unique value to the patient undergoing such devastating changes in self-perception and in the perception of others.

Finally, the fact that manic-depressive illness is so effectively controlled by a chemical treatment makes certain problems particularly difficult to manage without psychological interventions. Medication is the central treatment, not an adjunctive one, and from time to time lithium noncompliance becomes a major theme in the therapy of many patients. Confusion often arises because both lithium and the illness itself can affect cognition, perception, mood, and behavior. Concerns about being on medication in general and specific concerns about lithium are substantive psychotherapeutic issues. As we shall see later, these concerns about lithium derive from both the direct effects of lithium on the illness (depriving some patients of much sought-after "highs" and energy) and the side effects of the drug.

What, then, from a more general perspective, are a few of the potential advantages and disadvantages of combining psychotherapy with pharmacotherapy? For relevant studies we must turn to the related, but in many respects very different, field of drug-psychotherapy interactions in the treatment of unipolar depression. No comparable controlled studies exist for bipolar manic-depressive illness, partially because of reasons mentioned earlier (easier alliance of depression with verbal treatments, less need for restraints, and so on), and partially because of the longer period of widespread clinical availability of the tricyclic antidepressants, as opposed to lithium, in the United States (roughly twenty years instead of ten). Although lithium has been available for a much longer time in Europe, virtually all the drug-psychotherapy studies have been conducted in this country.

Klerman (1975) outlined several potential negative and positive drug-psychotherapy interactions. Particularly relevant to the treatment of bipolar patients would be the hypothesized positive effects of drug treatment on psychotherapy (increased accessibility of the patient, psychotherapeutically useful symptomatic changes such as increased memory, improved sleep, enchanced verbal skills, decreased distractibility, and so forth and positive effects of psychotherapy during treatment with drugs (more reliable patient attendance, increased compliance with the drug regimen). Weissman (1978), in her review of the controlled studies of antidepressants alone and in combination with psychotherapy, concluded that: (1) in ambulatory, unipolar depressed outpatients, the combination of antidepressant medications with psychotherapy (group, individual, or conjoint) was more efficacious than either treatment alone, and (2) there were no negative drug-psychotherapy interactions (findings further documented by Rounsaville, Klerman, and Weissman, 1981).

Analogous studies for the treatment of bipolar illness do not exist. Thus, in our discussions we shall be limited to more hypothetical issues, supplemented by a few noncontrolled clinical investigations. Several modalities of psychotherapy are available to the clinician wishing to work with patients who are taking lithium. Informal psychological treatments include the supportive role of the physician in medication management; the application of educational models conveying medical information about manic-depressive illness and lithium through lectures, hand-outs, films, or information-giving groups; and, finally, self-help groups, modeled on Alcoholics Anonymous, run by patients for themselves. A wide range of theoretical orientations govern more formal psychological treatments such as individual, group, family, and conjoint psychotherapy or some combination of these.

Very little is known about the appropriateness of any of these modalities, or orientation for any given patient and/or type of presenting problem. For example, it is not known whether cognitive-behavior therapy is more effective for lithium compliance problems and psychodynamic therapy more appropriate for the interpersonal sequelae of bipolar illness. Likewise, it is not known whether group therapy is more useful for problems of illness denial and of self-esteem and, relatedly, whether individual therapy is more appropriate for short-term crisis intervention (such as in suicidality) and/or long-term treatment of idiosyncratic, intrapsychic problems. There has been no research addressing these issues.

Clinical Reports of Combined Psychotherapy and Lithium Treatment

The lack of any systematic research on combined lithium treatment and psychotherapy limits our discussion to a small number of clinical reports (summarized in Table 5-1) and comments from anecdotal accounts. None of these studies focus on the interaction of individual psychotherapy with lithium. Only one of the clinical studies presented in the table uses comparison groups for the analysis of analyzing treatment outcome (Davenport et al., 1977), and only two of the remaining studies, one a continuation of the other (Shakir et at., 1979; Volkmar et al., 1980) use pre-and post-measures. The substantial methodological shortcomings in all of these investigations make data interpretations virtually impossible. However, the clinical observations made by the therapists conducting the studies are conceptually very useful.

TABLE 5-1 Clinical Reports of Combined Psychotherapy and Lithium Treatment

Author/ Year	Type of Therapy/ Therapeutic Orientation	Study Design/ Treatment Format	Patients	Results	Clinical Observations
Fitzgerald, 1972	*Family Therapy* and lithium eclectic: educational, emphasis on communications, playback of videotape sessions	Clinical study; no comparison group	N = 25 bipolar, index hospitalization for mania	No systematic follow-up	Family therapy can help manic patients: (1) continue to take lithium, (2) help prevent relapses, and (3) improve verbal communication within family system (that is, replace the role of mania in the expression of anger and frustration)
Davenport et al., 1977	*Couples Group Therapy* and lithium psychodynamic	Group I—Couples Group, therapy weekly	N = 12 bipolar patients and spouses	No rehospitalizations No marital failures	Family interactions and social functioning best in Couples Group therapy; family interaction better in NIMH maintenance group than in community-referred; no significant difference between latter two groups on social functioning
		Group II—NIMH OPD, lithium maintenance monthly; crisis treatment as needed	N = 11 bipolar patients	2 rehospitalized 5 marital failures	Strong recommendation for co-therapist model
		Group III—Referral back to community; community clinic or private care	N = 42 bipolar patients	16 rehospitalized 10 marital failures 3 suicides	Marital dynamics: (1) fear, by both partners, of recurrence; (2) sense of helplessness; (3) need to control all affect and defend against closeness; (4) use of massive denial; and (5) themes related to early parental loss and failure to grieve
		Note: Marriages intact at time of discharge from index hospitalization for all patients; follow-up period variable for all groups (2–10 years post-hospitalization)			

Shakir et al., 1979	*Group Therapy* and lithium interpersonal, interactional, "here and now"	Clinical study; compared group means of patients' pre/post hospitalization records. 75 minutes weekly. Lithium dispensed during last 30 minutes of group	N = 15 bipolar patients; 13 men, 2 women; mean age: 43; range: 19–63; mean duration on lithium prior to group: 21 months	*Pre-Group* 16 weeks/ year in hospital *Post-Group* 3 weeks/ year in hospital Two-year follow-up	Group themes: (1) initial skepticism about lithium and group therapy; (2) complaints of loss of well-being due to lithium; (3) denial of problems; (4) projected responsibility for lithium efficacy onto psychiatrist; (5) concerns: fears of recurrence, illness chronicity, social adjustment, and social acceptance
Rosen, 1980	*Group Therapy* and lithium directive	Clinical study; no comparison group of pre/post measures. 90 minutes every 4 weeks	N = 25 patients, mixed diagnoses; 12 men, 13 women; mean age: 36; range: 25–57.	No systematic follow-up; after 2 ½ years 8 patients remained in group	Group themes: (1) lithium, (2) concerns about manic-depressive illness, (3) lowered morale when a group member hospitalized; described lively group atmosphere where "therapist works not so much to stimulate interaction as to moderate it"
Volkmar et al., 1980	*Group Therapy* and lithium interpersonal, interactional, "here and now"	(Continuation of group therapy outlined in Shakir et al., 1979)			Group themes as reported in Shakir et al. above, additional comments: cessation of lithium use resulted in denial of illness, lack of information about lithium, and lack of support from family and friends: "It is not clear whether the high rate of compliance is secondary to the effects of group therapy per se or to the close follow-up the patients received or to the interaction between the two"

Common Psychotherapeutic Issues

Lithium is a unique drug in psychiatry; it is prophylactic and is both an antimanic and antidepressant agent. Paradoxically, at high blood levels, it can produce signs of both depression (lethargy, slowed speech, impaired cognition, apathy) and, less commonly, mania (a neurotoxicity-induced organic brain syndrome which can mimic or trigger mania). Finally, it is a maintenance medication which, to date, remains relatively free of the unfortunate side effects associated with the use of the phenothiazines and butyrophenones.

Ironically, because lithium is such a highly effective medication, there is a tendency for many therapists to minimize the value of their own role, and the role of psychotherapy, in the treatment of manic-depressive illness. Although there is little research on the subject, it should be kept in mind that many patients find psychotherapy a highly useful adjunct to lithium treatment. In one study (Jamison, Gerner, and Goodwin, 1979), twice as many patients as therapists thought that psychotherapy was valuable as an adjunct to lithium treatment.

Without question, the competent and compassionate psychotherapy of manic-depressive illness is predicated upon a solid knowledge of the illness. Kraepelin's (1904) injunction to his turn-of-the-century medical students remains a compelling one: "...it is one of the physician's most important duties to make himself, as far as possible, acquainted with the nature and phenomena of insanity." A solid knowledge of manic-depressive illness encompasses phenomenology; the natural history of the illness, including its cyclicity and degree of predictability; and biological aspects of the illness, including drug responses in mania and depression, biological theories of etiology, and mechanisms of actions of the drugs used in its treatment. A good scientific grasp of phenomenology and biology generally increases therapeutic self-assurance and decreases two problems common in less comprehensively trained therapists: (1) biological overdeterminism, often caused by therapists well-grounded in biological theories but poorly trained in psychological studies (for example, personality theory and development, perception, motivation, learning theory), and, (2) the tendency to ignore or downplay, or conversely to overemphasize, the biological substrate because of an inadequate understanding of it.

The psychotherapy of manic-depressive illness requires considerable flexibility in style and technique. This flexibility is necessitated by the changing moods, cognitions, and behaviors and fluctuating levels of dependency intrinsic to the illness. In the therapeutic relationship an overtly permissive approach is often useful to maximize the patient's sense of control of his behavior. It is important not to overcontrol the patient and not to allow lithium to become the focus of a power struggle. The symbolic value of lithium is enormous, and its role as a projective device is also extremely important (discussed below in greater detail). A thin line exists between overly extensive therapeutic control (which can lead to increased dependency, decreased self-esteem, decreased compliance, and increased acting-out) and too little control (occasionally leading to feelings of insecurity, unnecessarily tenuous holds on reality, and feelings of abandonment). Thus, firmness and consistency in ordering routine lithium levels or tests of thyroid and kidney functioning may be interpreted as caring, but undue emphasis on precise medication patterns (for example, not allowing for some degree of self-titration) may result in unnecessary power struggles and problems in lithium compliance. Collaborative aspects of management—self-ratings, chartings, patient and family education (through films, lectures, books, handouts)—are also an integral part of good clinical care. Finally, it is vital that the therapist be able to use hospitalization as an occasionally necessary adjunct to outpatient care without regarding hospitalization as a rejection or punishment of the patient or as an indication of therapeutic failure.

Psychotherapy Issues:

In manic-depressive illness, psychotherapy issues can be conceptualized as those that involve *losses* (realistic, symbolic, and unrealistic) and those that involve *general concerns* about the illness and its effect on the patient and his life.

1. *Realistic losses* are those regretted alterations of prior functioning because of the effects of lithium on the symptoms themselves. These changes can include decreases in energy level, loss of euphoric states, increased need for sleep, possible decreases in productivity and creativity, and decreased sexuality. (Jamison, Gerner, and Goodwin, 1979; Polatin and Fieve, 1971; Schou and Baastrup, 1973; Schou, 1980; Van Putten, 1975).

A recent study of patient attributions suggested that many patients felt their manic-depressive illness made positive contributions to their lives in one or more important ways, specifically, through increased sexuality, productivity, creativity, and sociability (Jamison et al., 1980). Attributions of such kinds are important for several reasons. From a clinical perspective it is important to realize the meaning, nature, and value of positive behavior and mood changes (as well as negative ones) for an individual patient. From a learning theory point of view, such altered states of consciousness during euthymic or depressed periods can be highly potent reinforcers that create in some patients a potentially strong, variable reinforcement schedule with significant benefits on the one hand and the risk of severe emotional and pragmatic problems on the other.

Treatment management under such circumstances is not an altogether straightforward matter. For example, compliance with a therapeutic lithium regime—which, at best, has a tenuous and delayed relationship with the alleviation of dysphoric features of manic-depressive illness—competes with a highly positive, intermittent reinforcement schedule, an exceedingly difficult behavior pattern to modify. In some ways it is analogous to a drug self-administration paradigm in which a highly pleasurable and often immediate state can be obtained. Thus, for some patients the illness may represent, in effect, an endogenous stimulant addiction. Clinical experience suggests that patients may attempt to induce mania by discontinuing lithium, not just at times when they are depressed, but also when they have to face problematic decisions and life events. Because the negative consequences accrue only later, it is understandable that it is not always clear to the patient that the costs outweigh the benefits.

Thus, it is important that the clinician be aware of the positive features of mood swings, to understand the nature of affective disorders better and thereby be more effective therapeutically, particularly with patients on lithium maintenance. The subtle and powerful clinician-patient alliance possible in lithium therapy is predicated on a thorough understanding of not only the benefits of lithium to the patient but also the realistic and unrealistic fantasies of loss that many patients have at some point before or during lithium treatment. These fantasies often focus on missing "highs" and cannot effectively be understood through simplistic formulations of the patient's being shortsighted, regressive, or escapist. Effective therapy with bipolar patients, whether it be drugs alone or a combination of drugs and psychotherapy, must address the reality of the patient's positive perceptions of the illness as well as the altered state of perception induced by phases of the illness.

Other losses consequent to being on lithium treatment include those in the patient's cognitive, perceptual, physical, emotional, or social spheres, which come about as a result of lithium side-effects, or social sequelae of having lithium therapy (for example, self-labeling or social stigma). The most significant side effects from a psychotherapeutic point of view are those detailed by Schou and Baastrup (1973) and Schou (1980): decreased energy, decreased enthusiasm and sexuality (occasionally a factor in increased marital problems), curbing of activities, and a commonly held perception that life is flatter and less colorful. Again, of course, it may be difficult to separate lithium side effects from the medication's impact on symptoms of the illness.

2. *Symbolic losses* can include a loss of perceived omnipotence and independence. Also, because of learned associations (the pairing of lithium with dysphoric states), lithium may symbolize a certain loss of innocence from a prepsychotic consciousness to a postpsychotic one. In this context lithium noncompliance can represent an attempt to recapture an earlier prepsychotic existence, one not yet "spoiled" by mania or depression.

3. *Unrealistic losses* include circumstances where lithium and psychotherapy come to symbolize the patient's personal failures. In addition to the normal difficulties in adjusting to the necessity for treatment, patients occasionally project all of their other life failures, thwarted ambitions, and inadequacies onto lithium. Under such circumstances, lithium can become the psychological whipping boy and represent a rationalization for other failures in the patient's life which existed before the onset of an affective disorder.

Therapeutic issues of general concern involve many areas of patients' adjustment to having manic-depressive illness: fears of recurrence, denial of the illness, discrimination of normal from pathological moods, effects of the illness on normal development tasks, and others. Let us look at a few of these in greater detail.

1. *Fears of recurrence* are almost ubiquitous in patients with manic-depressive illness. Some patients become preoccupied with such fears and are almost illness-phobic; they become unduly self-protective and hyperalert for signs of an impending episode. These concerns are often reflected in the process of learning to differentiate normal from abnormal moods and states. A related concern is a perceived decreasing tolerance for affective episodes. This is usually secondary to the stress of the illness and to the large amounts of psychological energy consumed by earlier bouts of depression and mania. Patients often express fears about the decreasing tolerance in their families and friends for such

recurrences. Bipolar illness also takes a severe toll in its *cumulative effects*. Thus Lowell (1977) wrote, "but the breakage can go on repeating once too often," and Logan (1976) described in his autobiography a certain weariness: "I was only forty-five years old, but I felt exhauted by this last experience, hollowed out, as though I were a live fish disemboweled."

2. *Denial of the illness*, of its severity, occasionally even of its existence, and of the possibility of recurrence are frequent clinical themes in bipolar illness. In some instances, the cognitive impairments in depression are sufficiently pronounced that they alone account for some problems in recollection. More often, repression and psychological and temporal distance cause the depression to pale into relative insignificance for a certain proportion of patients. Frequently, the severity and nature of the manic episode is minimized or "forgotten." Again, this can be due to several factors: the relatively clearer perception for the earlier and more enjoyable stages of mania, amnesia secondary to the organic features of manic psychosis, and repression; also, the sheer volume of cognitions, perceptions, and behaviors during mania make good recall unlikely.

Denial of the illness has been seen as crucial in lithium noncompliance by many researchers (Cade, 1949; Jamison, Gerner, and Goodwin, 1979; Polatin and Fieve, 1971; Schou et al., 1970; Van Putten, 1975). Our survey of the attitudes of fifty clinicians, each of whom had treated at least fifty patients with lithium, found that 64 percent of them felt that lithium noncompliance was a result of patients acting out their denial of a serious, lifelong illness (Jamison, Gerner, and Goodwin, 1979).

3. *Problems in learning to discriminate normal from abnormal moods* are common throughout the psychotherapy of bipolar patients maintained on a lithium regimen. Many manic-depressives, because of the intensity of their emotional responses, fear the escalation of a normal depressive reaction into a major depressive episode and, less commonly, fear the escalation of a state of well-being into hypomania or mania. Many emotions, of course, range into several mood states, spanning euthymia, depression, and hypomania. For example, irritability and anger can be a part of normal human existence or alternately can be symptoms of both depression and hypomania. Tiredness and lethargy can be due to normal circumstances, medical causes, or clinical depression as can sadness and pessimism. Feeling good, being productive, and enthusiastic, and working hard can be either normal, or pathognomonic of

hypomania. These overlapping emotions can be confusing and often arouse anxiety in many patients; these patients may then question their own judgment and become unduly concerned about recurrences of their affective illness. Occasionally, patients become conservative or excessively conforming. Benson (1974) notes that manic-depressives "tend to be more conservative and more conforming to others' attitudes because they are afraid that their ideas are the result of their misperception."

Therapy often consists of helping the patient discriminate normal from abnormal affect and of teaching him to live within a narrower range of emotions while learning to use those emotions with greater subtlety and discretion. Closely related to the discrimination of moods is the slow, steady process involved in patients' learning to unravel what is normal personality from what has been superimposed upon it in terms of turbulence, impulsiveness, lack of predictability, and depression. Of course, it takes a long period of time before adjustment, stabilization, and insight occur.

4. *Developmental tasks*, previously overshadowed by the manic-depressive illness, often become issues for the euthymic patient. In an ironic sense, manic-depressive illness can act in some ways as a protection against many of the slings and arrows of fortune encountered in normal life. Because late adolescence and early adulthood are the highest risk periods for the onset of the illness, many of the developmental tasks of these periods—individuation, interpersonal intimacy, romantic involvements, hurts, and rejections, and career developments—are impaired or temporarily halted. Once the illness is in remission and/or under control, patients often have to deal with these problems—as well as those of a more general, existential nature—within the therapeutic situation.

5. *Concerns about effects of the illness on a family system* can be profound. Patients often report feeling guilty about things done while in mania and those left undone in depression. The most frequently voiced concerns center on the interpersonal sequelae of the illness, generally effects felt by spouses, family members, and friends. Mayo, O'Connell, and O'Brien (1979) studied the families of twelve patients with manic-depressive illness and described the tremendous impact of the illness on the family system.

6. *Concerns about the genetic component* of manic-depressive illness are considerable for many patients. Such concerns relate to guilt over possible transmission of the disorder to children; overidentification and prob-

lems with individuation when a close family member, particularly a parent, has the illness; and, occasionally, guilt over receiving an effective treatment—lithium—which was not available to an afflicted parent. This latter phenomenon, although not common, is particularly striking in those patients whose parents either committed suicide or were hospitalized for long periods of time. A similar guilt is sometimes seen in those patients successfully treated with lithium whose siblings or parents refuse treatment.

Countertransference Issues

As we saw in an earlier section, many psychoanalysts who worked in the prelithium era found it a frustrating task to treat manic-depressive patients. Countertransference issues were openly discussed, and anger with such patients for their seeming inconstancy and lack of insight (or desire for same) was described in some detail. Spurgeon-English (1949) said succinctly what others said at great length: "The manic-depressive rejects you because he seems to be unsure that he needs you at all." Although many aspects of therapeutic work with manic-depressives have radically changed as a result of lithium, strong countertransference feelings continue to be elicited through such patients. Therapists who work with bipolar patients are often frustrated by inconsistencies in patient behavior and attitudes (toward self, therapist, therapy, lithium) during different mood states. These various moods and selves can result in fluctuating levels of intimacy and trust within the therapeutic relationship—both from patient to therapist and therapist to patient.

Anger and frustration can also be engendered in the therapist if a patient rejects an effective treatment; patient omnipotence can confront therapist omnipotence (reinforced by a highly potent medication) in a classic power struggle. Often the basis of such encounters is a lack of comprehension by the therapist of the meaning of the illness to the patient (as well as a lack of understanding on the part of the patient, usually secondary to denial, about the consequences of rejecting such a treatment regimen). Greenson (1967) emphasized the importance of an analyst with a broad and rich background for empathy; this breadth of fantasy is particularly relevant and useful to the therapist who deals with psychotic patients, who may allude to emotions and ideas foreign to the experiential base of the therapist. In addition to the kind of personal background advocated by Greenson, feelings of exclusion from this kind of experience can also be reduced by a solid grounding in phenomenology.

Therapists often experience anger and feelings of impotence when denial and omnipotence in the patient, leading to lithium noncompliance, result in rehospitalization for manic or depressive episodes, suicide attempts, or exacerbations in hostile and aggressive behaviors. Feelings of inadequacy and failure due to a recurrence of the illness can occur even if the patient is compliant; such feelings in the therapist often occur when treating any patient who is depressed, suicidal, or hypomanic (Fromm-Reichmann, 1949; Janowsky et al., 1970). For example, when hypomanic, a patient may show a special sensitivity to vulnerabilities in the therapist. Such awareness of, and tuning in to, the therapist's vincibility is the core of many acute, intense feelings of rage and violation by the therapist. Although this pattern of interaction is most likely to occur during hypomania and mania, it is not uncommon during the depressive phase when the patient's defenses are down and his level of paranoia, irritability, and hopelessness increases. Patients under such circumstances are often exquisitely tuned in to feelings of frustration, annoyance, and impotence in the therapist; anger and hopelessness expressed by the patient at such times often have a large impact on the already vulnerable therapist. In such instances, of course, the recognition of and effective coping with countertransference feelings are vital, so that the repercussions are minimal for the depressed patient.

Yet another problem with countertransference potential centers on misinterpretation of resistance when dealing with manic-depressive patients. We discussed earlier such patients' difficulties in differentiating normal from pathological mood states as well as their fears of recurrence. Occasionally therapists assume that a patient's depression is reactive to a particular environmental, interpersonal, or therapeutic event, and thus problems in discussing and handling that event are attributed to resistance. Often such depressions represent mild breakthrough cycling in the illness, which the patient senses but cannot articulate. The therapist's tendency to link such feelings with external events can be problematic. Even when the depressions are not really "endogenous," patients often are frightened by the similarity between such affects and cognitions and earlier, severe depressive episodes. A delicate therapeutic approach is needed both to help the patient in differentiating types of feelings and to assist the therapist in recognizing the possible need to deny recurrence or to see psychological causality where little exists.

Another area of potential countertransference problems concerns the therapist's acting-out through the patient. The therapist is in a unique position and can influence the patient—both through unconscious encouragement of behaviors linked to affective states and through unconscious encouragement of lithium noncompliance. Also of relevance is the special appeal of the illness in general and of hypomania and mania in particular. A potential exists for envy, projective identification, and seduction, as well as guilt over depriving patients of a special state (often heightened by patient resistance to lithium and proclaimed missing of "highs"). Unconscious collusion in medication resistance is not an uncommon problem. Likewise, the seductive aspects of hypomania are often impossible to ignore, and a therapist's seduced response can be illustrative of the reasons why patients miss their highs in the first place. Moods are obviously contagious, and occasionally the loss of a patient's hypomania results in a corresponding, albeit obviously lessened, loss reaction in the therapist as well. A certain number of psychotherapists espouse a set of attitudes about psychosis which we term the "Equus-Laingian view of madness." We refer to a romantization or erotization of madness which can range from a tendency to overvalue the positive aspects of manic-depressive illness while minimizing the negative, painful ones to a conviction that all psychopharmacological interventions in such patients are oppressive and contraindicated.

Lithium Compliance

With a growing number of patients receiving lithium therapy, a drug well established as useful in the treatment and prophylaxis of affective disorders, problems with compliance have become common. No data exist on how many patients actually stop taking lithium against medical advice, for what reasons and for how long, at what point in their therapeutic regime or mood cycles, and whether or not there are sex and age differences in the incidence of and reasons for noncompliance or incomplete compliance. Very little systematic research has been done on patients' perceptions of the positive and negative consequences of taking the drug regularly and on the effect of these perceptions on actual patterns of lithium use.

Several anecdotal reports of lithium noncompliance have been published, along with some proposed explanations for the phenomenon. Polatin and Fieve (1971) emphasized that patients often attribute decreases in creativity and productivity to lithium; the authors also stressed the role of lithium noncompliance in the denial of a chronic, serious illness. Fitzgerald (1972) speculated that refusal to take lithium stemmed from intolerance of reality-based depressions, preference for a hypomanic life style, or provocation by a spouse or other family member who also missed the patient's hypomanic episodes. Van Putten (1975) stresses the missing of hypomania by both patients and family members and states the importance of lithium side effects and lithium-induced dysphoria, characterized by a driveless, anhedonic condition (T. Van Putten, M.D., written communication, 1977). He, as do Schou et al. (1970), also mentions depressive relapse, as well as a tendency to feel well and to see no further need for medication, as significant variables in lithium refusal. Kerry (1978) suggested that the social stigmatization of manic-depressive illness may lead to rejection of the most concrete symbol of the illness.

In a preliminary exploration of these and related questions, we pursued two obvious sources of information and experience: the attitudes of patients themselves ($N = 47$ lithium patients from the UCLA Affective Disorders Clinic) and, independently, of clinicians well experienced in the use of lithium ($N = 50$ physicians, each of whom had treated at least fifty patients with lithium; many had treated hundreds more). We found it remarkable that nearly one-half (47 percent) of the patients reported having stopped lithium therapy at some time, against medical advice, and of those, 34 percent said that they stopped taking lithium more than once. Of those who reported that they had *not* stopped, over 90 percent stated they had never considered stopping, which suggests the possibility of two distinct subgroups of patients, a distribution perhaps more bimodal than continuous in nature. The results of the study are summarized below.

Demographic Results

No significant differences were found in sex, age, education, or income between the group of patients who reported that they discontinued lithium treatment against medical advice ($N = 22$) and the group of patients who did not ($N = 25$). Patients with a prior history of mania (bipolar I) tended to be less compliant than those with a prior history of hypomania (bipolar II). The number of months of lithium therapy was the only variable found that significantly differentiated the groups; more patients reported discontinuing lithium during long-term treatment. These preliminary data do not allow further inference about the increasing tendency to discontinue lithium over time; they may reflect only the effect of increasing the period at risk for noncompliance.

Perceived Effectiveness of Lithium

Both groups of patients reported lithium to be highly effective in the prevention of recurrences of mania and effective, although somewhat less so, in the prevention of recurrent depressions. Interestingly, 96 percent of the clinicians found lithium extremely or very effective treatment for mania, while 73 percent of the patients evaluated it as such, and more patients (40 percent) than clinicians (24 percent) regarded lithium as an effective treatment of depression. However, no significant relationship existed between perceived effectiveness and reported compliance.

Perceived Importance of Psychotherapy

In contrast to the patient group, 50 percent of whom considered psychotherapy to be "very important" in lithium compliance, only 27 percent of the clinicians (most of whom were practicing psychotherapists) regarded therapy as "very important." This may indicate a tendency for clinicians to value the potency of an effective medication so highly that they underestimate psychological aspects of the illness and medication compliance. However, more than half the clinicians (59 percent) indicated that they almost always encouraged patients to seek adjunctive psychotherapy.

Motivation for Continuing Lithium Treatment

Both the compliant and noncompliant patient groups indicated that a fear of depression was a stronger reason for staying on lithium than was a fear of mania. The clinicians concurred in this perception.

Side Effects of Lithium

Clinicians tended to rate side effects as more important factors in noncompliance than did those patients who reported discontinuing lithium therapy. Both patients and clinicians viewed lethargy, impairment in coordination, and lithium-induced tremor as the most important side effects in noncompliance. However, patients regarded dulling of senses as equally important to them, whereas clinicians emphasized weight gain. Interestingly, three of the four side effects seen as most important by clinicians (tremor, weight gain, nausea, and vomiting) are all relatively somatic or medical in nature, which may in part reflect a tendency for patients to mention physical rather than cognitive changes to their physicians. Conversely, it may be that clinicians are somewhat reluctant to acknowledge substantial cognitive changes, or perhaps they tend to view such changes as aspects of the affective illness rather than of the medication. Female patients regarded lethargy and dulling of senses as significantly more problematic than did male patients.

General Reasons for Noncompliance

Table 5–2 lists in rank order of importance the reasons cited by the entire patient sample, by the group who had reported noncompliance, and by the clinicians. A considerable agreement existed between patient and clinician perceptions, with a few significant exceptions. Patients were much more bothered by the idea that their moods were controlled by medication than the clinicians perceived them to be. Patients perceived lithium as being more effective in preventing depressions than did the clinicians and also felt, more strongly than did clinicians, that psychotherapy was important in helping them continue lithium treatment. From the patient's perspective, the most important reasons for noncompliance were: (1) a dislike of the idea that their moods were controlled by medication, (2) being bothered by the idea of having a chronic illness, symbolized by the necessity of lithium therapy, and (3) side effects, particularly lethargy, decreased coordination, and dulling of senses. Those patients who reported discontinuing lithium were also significantly more likely to report "missing highs" and the hassle of taking medications as important reasons for noncompliance. On the other hand, decreased productivity, creativity, and attractiveness to spouse or friends were generally perceived by patients as not very important

TABLE 5-2 Lithium Compliance

RANK ORDERS OF GENERAL REASONS FOR NONCOMPLIANCE

Total Patient Sample	*Patients Who Reported Discontinuing Lithium Treatment*	*Independent Clinician Sample*
1. Bothered by idea that moods are controlled by medication	Bothered by idea that moods are controlled by medication	Felt well, saw no need for lithium
2. Felt depressed	Missed "highs"*	Missed "highs"
3. Bothered by idea of chronic illness	Felt depressed	Bothered by idea of chronic illness
4. Felt less attractive to spouse	Bothered by idea of chronic illness	Felt less creative
5. Felt well, saw no need for lithium	Felt well, saw no need for lithium	Felt less productive
6. Hassle to take medications	Hassle to take medications*	Bothered by idea that moods are controlled by medication
7. Missed "highs"	Felt less attractive to friends	Hassle to take medications
8. Felt less creative	Felt less creative	Felt less attractive to friends
9. Felt less productive	Felt less productive	Felt depressed
10. Felt less attractive to friends	Felt less attractive to spouse	Felt less attractive to spouse

Source: Jamison, Gerner, and Goodwin, *Archives of General Psychiatry,* 1979.

* $p < .05$: patients who actually discontinued the lithium regime rated these reasons as significantly more important than did those patients who did not stop lithium therapy.

reasons for discontinuing lithium. This is in contrast to several prevailing notions about reasons for noncompliance and suggests that "highs" are not necessarily equated with creativity or productivity by most patients.

From the clinician's point of view, the most important reasons for lithium noncompliance were: (1) the patient felt well and saw no need to continue the medication; (2) the patient missed the "highs" of hypomania; and (3) the patient was bothered by the idea of having a chronic illness.

There were no significant differences by sex in the rate of noncompliance. In terms of side effects, women were significantly more concerned with perceived lethargy and dulling of senses than were men; it is possible that women are more sensitive or bothered by these effects for psychosocial reasons or that hormonal changes produce subtle changes in lithium retention that result in more subtoxic episodes of symptom exacerbation. Although in this relatively small sample there were no overall significant differences in scores between men and women on general reasons for noncompliance, women were more likely to mark "missing highs" and "being bothered by the idea of their moods being controlled by medication" as very important. One could speculate that women may perceive more desirable benefits from their "highs" than do men because of more extensive changes from baseline experience (such as hypersexuality, increased energy, and productivity); some corroborating evidence for this hypothesis has been presented (Jamison et al, 1980). Too, women may be more accustomed to accepting extremes of moods and emotions as being within the bounds of normal feminine behavior and culturally sanctioned experience and, consequently, may be more upset by the idea of external control. It is possible that, as a result of the natural history of bipolar illness, women may experience more frequent mini-affective episodes, leading to more accommodation of such mood swings, if not to actual acceptance and learned modulation. Men, on the other hand, may regard fluctuating moods as more aberrant and thus more legitimately subject to external or medical control. Although not systematically studied, the legal and financial sequelae may be more extensive for men than for women, because of differences in cultural expectations and in actual phenomenology of the illness (for example, men's higher ratio of mania to depressive episodes, more aggressive and destructive behavior when manic, and greater physical strength). In short, it is probable that the cost-benefit ratio of lithium compliance is different for men and women.

Psychodynamic Issues

More than one-half the physicians (64 percent) felt that lithium noncompliance was "somewhat" or "very" related to patients acting out their denial of having a serious lifelong illness. Thirty-five percent of the clinicians felt that, by not complying, patients were acting out psychodynamic factors in therapy. Approximately one-fourth (26 percent) felt that patient anger directed toward the therapist or a significant other was also an important reason for patients to discontinue lithium therapy against medical advice.

It is clear from our findings, and from those of others, that incomplete compliance with lithium is a major clinical problem and one that brings with it a substantially increased risk of personal and interpersonal chaos, hospitalization, and suicide. Approximately one-half of our patients reported discontinuing lithium treatment against medical advice at least once. On the basis of extensive clinical experience, the physicians in our sample estimated that one-third of those patients taking lithium would stop taking it against medical recommendations. These figures are consistent with other reports in the literature; Van Putten (1975), in his review, summarized available statistics and concluded that 20 to 30 percent of patients with manic-depressive illness discontinue their lithium treatment against medical advice. It is again interesting to note that, of the thousands of lithium citations in the scientific literature, only a few papers (those discussed in an earlier section) focused on the psychological or psychotherapeutic aspects of lithium treatment.

One more relevant detail should be mentioned in the context of psychotherapy, lithium, and compliance—reinforcement schedules intrinsic to lithium treatment. Psychotherapy must contend with a singularly difficult set of problems in this regard: (1) lithium is a drug with delayed therapeutic action (five to seven days for an antimanic effect, three to five weeks for an antidepressant one); (2) it has no known reinforcing qualities, either immediate or delayed; (3) patients are expected to stay on the drug for indeterminate periods of time, most of it in a euthymic state (and therefore without symptomatic motivation); (4) if a patient stops the medication, the negative consequences of noncompliance (that is, recurrence of the affective illness) are almost always long-delayed in time, providing no immediate negative reinforcer; (5) the onset of the initial lithium treatment is often paired with highly aversive emotional states (depression, mania, dysphoria); (6) if the initial lithium is prescribed for a manic episode, the natural history of the illness predicts that any given patient is at significant risk for a substantial post-mania depression; this further pairs the onset of lithium treatment with dysthymia; and (7) the cessation of lithium is often accompanied by relatively immediate positive experiences, either due to the disappearance of side effects or to the experience of breakthrough hypomanias (often a contributing factor in lithium noncompliance).

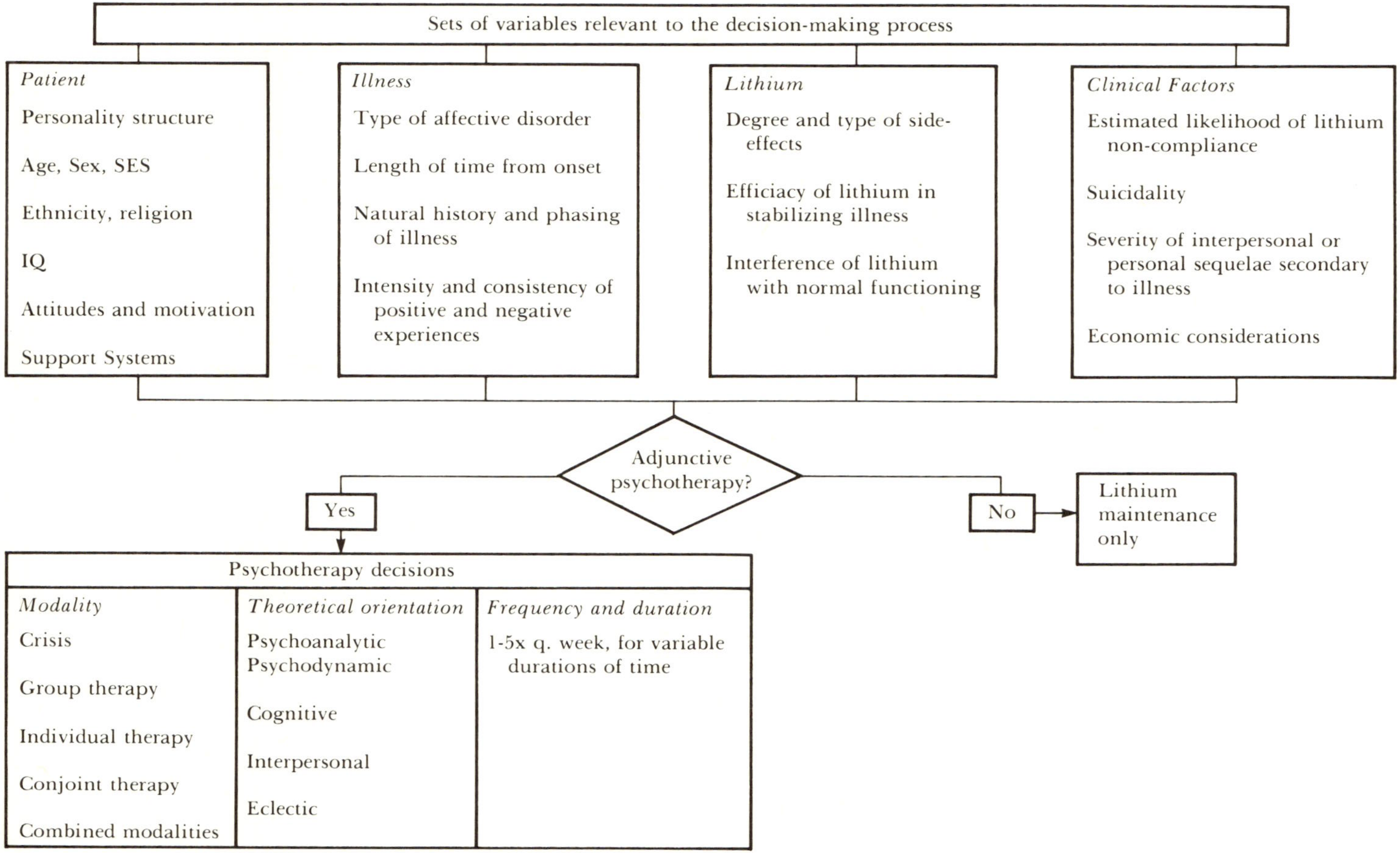

Figure 5–1. Adjunctive psychotherapy in the lithium patient: variables in the decision-making process.

References

ABRAHAM, K. Notes on the psychoanalytic investigation and treatment of manic-depressive insanity and allied conditions. In *Selected papers of Karl Abraham.* London; Hogarth Press, 1968.

BENSON, R. The forgotten treatment modality in bipolar illness: Psychotherapy. *Dis. Nerv. Sys. 35:*634–638, 1974.

——. Psychotherapy in bipolar illness. Unpublished manuscript.

BUNNEY, W.E., JR., HARTMANN, E.L., and MASON, J.W. Study of a patient with 48-hour manic-depressive cycles. II. Strong positive correlation between endocrine factors and manic defense patterns. *Arch. Gen. Psychiat. 12:*619–625, 1965.

CADE, J.F.J. Lithium salts in the treatment of psychotic excitement. *Med. J. Aust. 2:*349–352, 1949.

DAVENPORT, Y.B., ELBERT, M.H., ADLAND, M.L., et al. Couples group therapy as an adjunct to lithium maintenance of the manic patient. *Amer. J. Orthopsychiat. 47:*495–502, 1977.

ENGLISH, O.S. Observation of trends in manic-depressive psychosis. *Psychiatry, 12:*125–134, 1949.

FITZGERALD, R.G. Mania as a message: Treatment with family therapy and lithium carbonate. *Amer. J. Psychother. 26:*547–555, 1972.

FROMM-REICHMANN, F. Intensive psychotherapy of manic-depressives. *Confina Neurologica, 9:*158–165, 1949.

JAMISON, K.R., GERNER, R.H., and GOODWIN, F.K. Patient and physician attitudes towards lithium. *Arch. Gen. Psychiat. 36:*866–869, 1979.

JAMISON, K.R., GERNER, R.H., HAMMEN, C., et al. Clouds and silver linings: Positive experiences associated with the primary affective disorders. *Amer. J. Psychiat. 137:*198–202, 1980.

JANOWSKY, D.S., LEFF, M., and EPSTEIN, R.S. Playing the manic game: Interpersonal maneuvers of the acutely manic patient. *Arch. Gen. Psychiat. 22:*252–261, 1970.

JENNER, F.A., and EASTWOOD, P.R. Renal effects of lithium. In Johnson, F.N. and Johnson, S. (Eds.), *Lithium in Medical Practice.* Baltimore; University Park Press, 1978, pp. 247–263.

JOHNSON, F.N. Social and psychological supportive measures during lithium therapy. In Johnson, F.N., (Ed.), *Handbook of lithium therapy.* Lancaster; MTP Press Limited, 1980, pp. 248–254.

KERRY, R.J. Recent developments in patient management. In Johnson, F.N., and Johnson, S., (Eds.), *Lithium in Medical Practice.* Baltimore; University Park Press, 1978, pp. 337–353.

KRAEPELIN, E. *Lectures on Clinical Psychiatry.* London; Balliere, Tindall, and Cox, 1904.

MAYO, J.A., O'CONNELL, R.A., and O'BRIEN, J.D. Families of manic-depressive patients: Effect of treatment. *Amer. J. Psychiat. 136:*1535–1539, 1979.

PAVAN, F. and BEZOARI, M. Patient-therapist relationship during the institution of lithium salts treatment in manic-depressive psychosis. *Psihofarmakologija, 3:*353–356, 1974.

POLATIN, P., and FIEVE, R.R. Patient rejection of lithium carbonate prophylaxis. *J. Amer. Med. Assoc. 218:*864–866, 1971.

RADO, S. The problem of melancholia. *Int. J. Psychoanal. 9:*420–438, 1928.

ROSENFELD, H. Notes on the psychological and psychoanalytic treatment of depressive and manic depressive patients. In Azima, H., and Glueck, B.C. (Eds.), *Psychiatric research report 17.* Washington, D.C.; The American Psychiatric Association, 1963, pp. 73–83.

ROUNSAVILLE, B.J., KLERMAN, G.L., and WEISSMAN, M.M. Do psychotherapy and pharmacotherapy for depression conflict? Empirical evidence from a clinical trial. *Arch. Gen. Psych. 38:*24–29, 1981.

SCHOU, M. Social and psychological implications of lithium therapy. In Johnson, F.N. (Eds.), *Handbook of lithium therapy.* Lancaster: MTP Press Limited, 1980, pp. 378–381.

——, and BAASTRUP, P.C. Personal and social implications of lithium maintenance treatment. In Ban, T.A., Boissier, J.R., Gessa, G.J., et al, (Eds.), *Psychopharmacology, sexual disorders and drug abuse.* Amsterdam and London; North Holland, 1973, pp. 65–68.

——BAASTRUP, P.C., GROF, P., et al. Pharmacological and clinical problems of lithium prophylaxis. *Brit. J. Psychiat. 116:*615–619, 1970.

SHAKIR, S.A., VOLKMAR, F.R., BACON, S., et al. Group psychotherapy as an adjunct to lithium maintenance. *Amer. J. Psychiat. 136:*455–456, 1979.

VAN PUTTEN, T. Why do patients with manic-depressive illness stop their lithium? *Comp. Psychiat. 16:*179–182, 1975.

VOLKMAR, F.R., SHAKIR, S.A., BACON, S., et al. Group therapy as an adjunct to lithium maintenance. Paper presented to the American Psychiatric Association, San Francisco, 1980.

WEISSMAN, M.M. Psychotherapy and its relevance to the pharmacotherapy of affective disorders: From ideology to evidence. In Lipton, M.A., Di Mascio, A., Killam, K.F. (Eds.), *Psychopharmacology: A generation of progress.* New York; Raven Press, 1978: pp. 1313–1321.

CHAPTER 6

The Influence of Psychiatric Drug Therapy on the Future of Psychoanalysis

Mortimer Ostow

THE USE OF THERAPEUTIC CHEMICAL AGENTS permits us to see psychic phenomena in an entirely new dimension. Psychiatric drug therapy creates therapeutic experiments which offer the opportunity for wholly new observations. We can observe hitherto unknown correlations among clinical states, parameters of psychic function that respond to and resist drug therapy, and how the process of pathogenesis can be influenced. These data demand a review of many concepts of clinical psychiatry and psychoanalytic theory. The primary purpose of this chapter is to present some of the observations I have made and to suggest how they can influence current thinking. We shall briefly consider the influence of drug therapy upon psychoanalytic practice.

Given the introduction of a rapid, effective, and inexpensive drug therapy for mental illness, one would expect it to compete with psychoanalysis for patients. In fact, the recent decrease in demand for psychoanalytic treatment is often attributed to the availability of drug therapy. While it may be true that a few patients who might profit from analysis will be discouraged from undertaking it because of successful drug treatment, I believe that drug therapy offers more to the discipline than it takes away. There can be no doubt that drug therapy is utterly ineffective in treating classical neurosis. A large share of the responsibility for the decreasing demand for psychoanalytic treatment is attributable to the decreasing incidence of classical neurosis. Drug therapy does not compete with analysis in this area. (I am ignoring the usefulness of the newer sedatives, often called minor tranquilizers, in alleviating anxiety, unhappiness, and insomnia; these are useful for muting symptoms, but they do not undo illness.) Personality disorders which are also responsive to analysis are not, for the most part, helped by psychiatric drug treatment. On the other hand, the conditions for which drug therapy is most effective, namely depressive illness, mania, and schizophrenic episodes, are not classical indications for analysis. Psychiatric drug treatment may be considered inimical to analysis in that it contributes to the current expectation and demand that mental illness be treated quickly and efficiently, as it often can be with skillfully administered drug treatment.

Psychiatric drug therapy permits the analyst to treat patients who were unavailable and unresponsive previously. Perhaps the commonest situation is that of the patient who was accepted for treatment on the assumption that the diagnosis was neurosis or personality disorder and then, during the course of treatment, becomes clearly depressed. In the presence of depression, psychoanalytic treatment becomes all but impossible. While the transference may offer the patient some support, there is relatively little that the analyst can actively do to alleviate the illness. The successful introduction of drug treatment will relieve the patient, rescue the treatment, and strengthen the transference.

The same holds true for the less frequent schizophrenic or manic regression. But if that can be done for the regressions which occur *during* treatment, there is no reason why a patient cannot be accepted for treatment in a schizophrenic, manic, or depressive state, helped to recover from this episode by chemotherapy and psychotherapy, and then, in a state of remission, accepted into full, conventional psychoanalytic treatment.

To be sure, another parameter in the determination of psychic function is thereby added—the medication. It complicates the transference and the constellation of psychodynamic forces, but it also offers information not previously available or confirms what has previously only been suspected.

CASE 1: A young woman was accepted for treatment after discharge from a hospital following recovery from her second known acute schizophrenic attack. She was taking a large dose of tranquilizing medication which slowed her thinking and movement and imposed a parkinsonian cast to her appearance. She was seen three times a week. The first month or so of treatment was occupied with reassuring her against the possibility of imminent relapse, investigating superficially and reconstructing the dynamics of her breakdown and of her current clinical state, and helping her to reorient herself about social life, parents, and career. Simultaneously, the dose of medication was carefully decreased to the point where she began to relapse; it was then increased again but only to the dose necessary to protect her, a dose considerably lower than that given to her in the hospital.*

The treatment was then pursued with classical psychoanalytic technique: couch, free association, transference interpretation, dream interpretation, and recapture of early memories and relating them to the stresses which preceded *past* breakdowns and to *current* stresses. In the face of new stresses, an attempt was made to help the patient master them with analytic interpretations alone. If she could not, and showed early signs of relapse, the dose of medication was increased very slightly. When she mastered the stress, the dose was decreased again. In each instance the stress could be identified and it was understood how it elicited symptoms, their significance, and what the change in medication achieved. The same psychodynamic constellations that in illness created delusions in drug-controlled remission elicited only transparent fantasies. In every respect the patient has improved to a state as good as, and in some ways much better than, the mental state that had prevailed before her breakdown. She has embarked upon and is successfully pursuing a new career at a level much above her earlier aspirations and is at peace with the world.

*It should be noted that when drug therapy is administered along with psychoanalysis or intensive psychotherapy, it can be much more subtle and more finely regulated than when it is administered alone. Because the therapist sees the patient so frequently and is so intimately familiar with the daily fluctuations in moods and attitudes, the psychoanalyst can titrate the medication so that no more than the smallest effective dose is given, thereby minimizing side effects and sustaining the patient in a state as close to natural equilibrium as possible. I have often observed that an optimal antipsychosis therapeutic effect will be obtained with a dose of tranquilizing medication just less than that which will produce the extrapyramidal side effects.

Beyond a few general remarks, I do not wish to discuss the *technique* involved in combining drug therapy with psychotherapy and psychoanalysis. In most instances normal psychoanalytic procedure can be followed in conjuction with the administration of drugs. Obviously the act of prescribing drugs is a form of intervention by the analyst, and its meaning to the patient must be analyzed as an aspect of transference. Accepting medication from the analyst means entering into an object relation with him; it means to the patient letting himself trust the analyst. When the transference becomes negative, there will be resistance against taking the medication.

Taking medication may reinforce hypochondriacal tendencies in either of two ways. The patient frequently interprets the need to use chemical agents as an indication that his illness is organic rather than psychogenic. He understands this distinction to mean that his illness is permanent rather than reversible. Second, the side effects that frequently occur, especially with the tricyclic antidepression drugs, may be used as a reality nucleus for hypochondriacal fantasies.

A more general response by the patient relating to the administration of medication by the analyst is lowered self-esteem. Hypochondria may be considered a special instance of diminished self-esteem, in that the medication may be seen as contributing to reduce the patient's somatic self-esteem. Moreover, the patient may also feel that his psychic integrity and mental competence are undermined by the medication and thus unreliable. It is important to respect the patient's need for self-respect and for continuity in his identity feelings. This can be done by making medication changes as infrequently as possible, by carefully explaining to the patient the need for each change at the time that the change is recommended, and by permitting the patient to experience at least a normal range of mood swings without being expected to accept corrective changes in medication.

The very effectiveness of the medication can lead both patient and analyst to see it as a kind of magic. Such a view can be hazardous for both analyst and patient in a number of ways. The patient who is suffering and wants prompt relief can see the medication aspect of the combined therapy as much more important than the analysis. The patient who is no longer acutely ill may resent the organic implications of medication, unrealistically minimize its role, and expect too much of the analytic procedure. Even the most conscientious and dedicated analyst may find himself seduced by the rapid and profound changes produced by medication and may find himself distracted from the analytic aspect of the treatment.

What can be expected of combined treatment? When I first started combined treatment, twenty-five years ago, I entertained the hope that good analysis might make it possible for the patient ultimately to do without medication. Some patients do, in fact, require medication only for the initial attack in which they are treated and thereafter can do without it because of the therapeutic effect of the analysis. Most patients, however, are not so fortunate; they require medication either continuously or recurrently for major portions of their lives. This finding should not come as a surprise in view of our assumption of a constitutional vulnerability to the serious illnesses which defy analysis, schizophrenia and manic-depressive illness, and our experience that episodes of illness are less a matter of unusually intense traumata than they are of mild trauma upsetting a fragile equilibrium in a highly conflicted personality. In these vulnerable individuals, medication can be depended upon to prevent relapse in response to stress while the analysis helps the patient to find a reasonable and maximally gratifying modus vivendi within the options and restraints offered by external obstacles and by those internal inhibitions that cannot be overcome by analysis. Neither drug therapy alone nor analysis alone would be able to achieve this. Drug therapy can only undo a regression; overcoming a developmental arrest requires good psychotherapy.

Two related questions naturally come to the mind of the classical analyst in any such discussion: It is proper to give medication in the course of an analytic procedure? Can the combined procedure described here really be called analysis? Both questions are actually different aspects of a third question: Can one administer medication within a psychoanalytic treatment regimen without thereby compromising the analytic quality of the patient's treatment?

Depending upon what one emphasizes, different answers to this question are possible. My own view is that the combined treatment satisfies all the criteria for authentic analysis except for the requirement that the analyst play no "real" role in the patient's life, that is, that his role be restricted to analyzing. It is generally understood, however, that this noninvolvement is a goal, toward which one strives, rather than an actuality. The analyst cannot help playing a "real" role in the patient's life: when he requires financial compensation for his services; when he requires firm and binding time commitment from the patient; when he restricts the patient's choice of vacation schedule; when he recommends medical consultation for investigation of a physical symptom; when he abandons the patient who becomes depressed or psychotic in the course of psychoanalytic treatment, sending him to a nonanalytic psychiatrist or to a hospital; or when he withholds drug therapy from such a patient in the interest of preserving the "purity" of the analysis.

Nonetheless, it is important to emphasize that, for analysis to continue, the patient's responses to all his "real" relations with the analyst must be analyzed in respect to transference. Accordingly, I see no reason why the coordinated administration of medication requires that the treatment be excluded from the category of psychoanalysis.

My conclusion is that rather than offering a competitive threat, drug therapy offers new opportunities for the psychoanalyst, for psychoanalysis, and, most important, for patients subject to manic-depressive and schizophrenic illness.

Significant as drug therapy is for the practice of psychoanalysis, it is even more important as a source of new information. Administration of medication influences psychic states, so that each therapeutic endeavor becomes, in a sense, an experimental procedure. While the practicing psychiatrist is primarily interested in treating his patient, his efforts to do so yield information about both the patient and drug treatment in general. The influence of therapeutic chemicals upon psychic states is far from being completely explored. I shall present here some of my own observations, which I believe have both theoretical and practical significance, but for which validation is still required.

Some of my observations pertain broadly to psychiatry rather than to the narrow area of psychoanalysis. I shall present these first and will consider three different clinical states: schizophrenia, manic-depressive illness, and depression.

Schizophrenia is conventionally designated as paranoid, catatonic, or hebephrenic, as though these were separate and distinct varieties of the illness, though it is acknowledged that the symptoms of one form frequently appear in other forms of the illness. Many psychiatrists propose that schizophrenia is not a single illness and that the term as currently used refers to a number of different illnesses with overlapping symptoms.

Although my experience with schizophrenia is limited, I have observed that under the influence of tranquilizers or antidepression agents or combinations of these in varying doses, the form of schizophrenia may change from any one of these three categories to either of the other two. Patients do seem to prefer one of these states to the other two and, left without treatment, will revert to that state. Yet under the influence of these chemical agents, the manifestations of the illness can in many cases change to the extent that a psychiatrist who is unaware that medication has been used would make a different diagnosis. I believe that with careful observation, one could ascertain the general rule that governs these drug-induced changes.

The existence of some kind of relation between schizophrenia and depression has been made clear. Bleuler described such combinations in his classic textbook; our current nomenclature (DSM III) includes several categories which recognize the concurrence of schizophrenic and affective features.

More recently, a number of psychiatrists have commented on the fact that some patients, recovering from schizophrenia, seem to lapse unaccountably into depression. Two explanations have been offered. First, the depression is the patient's reaction to the same stress that precipitated the schizophrenic breakdown and appears now, after drug therapy has made schizophrenic illness unavailable as an escape. Second, the depression is the consequence of the action of the antischizophrenia tranquilizer. I believe that both of these views are correct, that is, both mechanisms may combine to elicit post-schizophrenia depression. However, I believe that the relation between schizophrenia and depression is more complex, and the specific problem of post-schizophrenia depression reflects only one aspect of it.

Among schizophrenic patients, one can distinguish two types: those relatively susceptible to depression and those relatively immune to it. The distinction is made all too easily in the course of drug therapy. Patients who recover relatively easily with medication and without complications are probably not susceptible to depression. Patients who become depressed on therapeutic doses of tranquilizer, or who become more severely psychotic, are susceptible to depression. If one wishes to obtain a remission in the patients of the latter class, one must combine antidepression with tranquilizing drug therapy. This can be done by careful titration, and the results can be very good. From a theoretical point of view, this observation has implications for brain chemistry; it is interesting that these two classes of drugs exert almost exactly opposite actions, yet they may be used simultaneously without canceling out each other's influence. The titration is theoretically easy but practically difficult because the tranquilizing drugs begin to work after a latency of twelve to twenty-four hours, while the antidepression drugs usually require an interval of three or four weeks before they become active. Observing such patients during the course of titration, one learns that either too much tranquilizer or too much energizer will make the patient more psychotic; remission is obtained only when tranquilizer and energizer are combined in a definite ratio. The clinical picture of tranquilizer-induced relapse and antidepression-induced relapse resemble each other in many ways, but differ in others. In the former instance one can usually note tell-tale indications of depression behind the schizophrenic symptoms. These include a preoccupation with death, hypochondria, guilt, a sense of letdown, a loss of "energy," and a feeling of aging rapidly. While the two states can be distinguished easily after one has seen both in the same patient, when initially confronted by one, it is often difficult to ascertain whether it is a "high" state or a "low" state.

In summary, I would draw the following inferences: schizophrenic and manic-depressive illness are seen in combination fairly frequently. Many schizophrenic patients, when first seen, are actually exhibiting such a combination. If the patient exhibits a "high" form of schizophrenia, he will respond easily to tranquilizing agents. If he is schizophrenic and depressed, tranquilizing agents will make him worse. If he is schizophrenic and vulnerable to depression, tranquilizing agents will produce an initial improvement which will then be followed by relapse.

Let us consider the struggle against depression. I have observed that a breakdown into definitive melancholic depression is frequently preceded by one or more of the following clinical states: First, the patient exhibits a state of paradoxic hypermotivation, that is, a state of unusual activity, sometimes presenting as mania or hypomania, sometimes as more limited activity, although it always has a "driven" quality to it. Denial is the characteristic defense of this state. Second, the patient is in a state of clinging attachment to an object who is regarded as a parent. This attachment is frequently expressed by subordinating oneself to the object and by deferring to the superego. The patient expresses regret and guilt for the previous acting out. Third, the patient exhibits a state of angry withdrawal from all objects, especially from the objects to whom the patient had previously clung for support, and, if the patient is in treatment, from the therapist. Detachment in one form or other characterizes this state.

When more than one of these states appear before the onset of depression, they appear in the order given. Each state may last hours, days, weeks, months, or years. Each state seems intended to combat a depressive tendency, the first by denial and substitute gratification, the second by dependence upon a mother substitute, and the third by narcissistic withdrawal. When one maneuver fails to retard the growing depressive tendency, it gives way to the next, or directly to the definitive depression. This sequential struggle against depression can sometimes be observed in the course of long-term psychoanalytic treatment.

If not regarded skeptically, the state of paradoxic hypermotivation may be interpreted as improvement. Similarly, the state of clinging dependence which frequently leads the patient to make an effort to please the analyst may be interpreted as a phase of increased insight. This interpretation offers a reason why some patients who seem to be doing especially well in treatment will suddenly and surprisingly lapse into depression.

Drug treatment makes the observation of this sequence fairly easy. These different states are often encountered when antidepression medication is withdrawn from a patient who requires its protection. It is frequently encountered when a tranquilizing drug is administered to a patient prone to manic-depressive fluctuations, as in the treatment of the hypomanic or the schizophrenic. In the latter case, the schizophrenic symptoms may obscure to some extent these antidepression states. If one is aware that the two illnesses may be combined, often enough the manifestations of each can be recognized. More convincing is the fact that drug treatment can influence those states which express the struggle against depression. If they truly represent this struggle, then they should be eliminated with antidepression treatment; in fact, they are. The paradoxical nature of the state of paradoxic hypermotivation is clearly revealed by the fact that it can be dissipated by an antidepression drug. In my experience, an antidepression drug will usually protect against mania as well as against depression.

Paradoxical hypermotivation may also activate a schizophrenic diathesis. In such cases the schizophrenic episode may be terminated by antidepression treatment with or without tranquilizing medication. One common manifestation of the state of clinging dependence is the appearance of phobic anxiety when the patient is separated from his anaclitic object; such phobias can be eliminated by antidepression drug therapy. The state of angry withdrawal may be represented in the neurotic individual by a hysterical withdrawal and in the psychotic by catatonic withdrawal. Such patients will respond well and promptly to antidepression medication.

Introducing chemical agents that influence psychic variables is likely to create some syndromes which do not appear naturally and to reproduce some syndromes which do occur naturally. One syndrome that does occur naturally, but under clinically diverse conditions so that its identity under these several conditions is not recognized, is the syndrome that I have called narcissistic tranquility. It comprises the following clinical findings: increased appetite; increased weight gain, more than commensurate with the increased intake; increased fluid retention; afternoon or evening torpor; increased sexual desire, which in the absence of an appropriate object, leads to frequent masturbation; and a tendency to acquire possessions. Narcissistic tranquility usually occurs when a patient remains under psychic stress but is protected from its traumatic effect by a counteractive force such as therapeutic medication, electric shock treatment, or the invoking of massive denial.

I consider the state of narcissistic tranquility a response to minor stress. The minor response contrasts with the major stress response, or the General Alarm Reaction of Selye, that is characterized by decreased appetite, weight loss, decreased sexual interest, and general arousal. I suspect that the former is associated with an increase in the mineralocorticoid to glucocorticoid ratio. It is of no serious consequence except that many patients become distressed at the inevitable weight gain and their inability to restrict eating. When this occurs, it is important that the analyst recognize it for what it is and understand that it implies the persistence of the struggle to maintain libidinal equilibrium. I know of no way to overcome the syndrome.

Let us turn now to observations more narrowly germane to psychoanalytic theory. One of the most striking and important observations made by everyone who uses drug therapy is the fact that certain components of mental function are readily affected by drug treatment and others are not. Obviously those components that do not change must be considered fixed, internal, and relatively permanent features of the personality. In current psychoanalytic language they are said to be crystallized into "structure." Those components that do change in response to medications recover from regression induced by disease. The following case study should illustrate these observations.

> Case 2: A married woman, twenty-eight years old, was first seen in a state of psychotic depression. While improvement was obtained within a few days with the use of small doses of Navane, a more effectively stabilizing formula of medication could not be worked out in less than six weeks. During that period of drug titration there were days when, under the influence of a formula that was too heavily weighted with antidepression medication, she became panicky, felt that her mind was leaving her body, and feared that she might be unable to control her suicidal impulse. On

other days, the formula was too heavily weighted by tranquilizing medication. She then felt inert, miserable, and afraid that she was losing her mind and was preoccupied with death. In both states she was preoccupied with death and concerned with what was happening to her mind. In the panicky state, she considered leaving her husband and children as she had in a previous psychotic episode. In the depressed state, she expressed guilt and wished to devote herself completely to the service of her family. When not psychotic in either way, she cultivated a concern with the meaning of life, whether there is life after death, whether she is a reincarnation of an individual from past generations, and how her soul would survive past her death. In childhood, she had attempted to deal with her profound difficulty in object relations and low self-esteem by narcissistic withdrawal and fairly transparent derivatives of a death wish. These mechanisms were clearly represented in both variants of her psychotic illness, the "high" variant and the depressed variant. What was different about these two psychotic states was the fear that she was about to detach from reality (that her mind was leaving her body, and an eagerness to escape from home and family) in the former state, and a guilty determination to subordinate herself to husband and children in the latter. What was common to the two and to the remission state must be considered fixed, developmentally crystallized components of her personality, while the variable features are the results of regression. The variables are more characteristic of the acute illness than of the personality.

This distinction between the fixed mechanisms, fantasies, and defenses specific to the individual and the changing and reversible symptoms characteristic of the illness must be taken into account in any modern psychoanalytic psychology.

The distinction between fixed and variable components of personality helps us to understand why neurosis and personality disorder can both resist drug therapy. At times, confronted with severely inhibited patients with personality disorders, I have attempted to mobilize them with antidepression medication in the hope that they might be helped to overcome their inhibitions. With this method, I found that I could intensify the level of activity but was unable to stimulate it sufficiently to permit them to overcome inhibitions. In addition to becoming active, they also became more belligerent, irritable, and often psychotically paranoid, using anger and projection to defend their inhibited state. In other instances I have used antidepression medication to treat the unhappiness of these inhibited patients. In these cases I was not treating classical melancholic depression but rather trying to induce a mild euphoria in order to relieve their desperation. Again, the improvement in mood often did not appear; when it did, it led to little improvement in functional capacity. When mood improvement did not appear, belligerence, irritability, and paranoia did.

The problem of assessing the "strength of the ego," in fact the problem of understanding the meaning of the term, has been studied by many analysts. It seems clear that strength and weakness cannot be considered points on any unidimensional scale. The phenomena that I have just described point to one dimension of ego strength that can easily be measured, that is, the resistance of the ego to the influence of tranquilizers and antidepression drugs. One may say that the patient who succumbs readily to depression with small doses of tranquilizing drugs displays a form of ego weakness. The same would be true in the case of the patient who responds readily with euphoria and overactivity to antidepression drugs. A different dimension of ego weakness is exhibited by the patient who, under the influence of these drugs, exhibits not only a mood change and shift in energy level but also responds with psychotic disorganization. Obviously, this proposition must be considered and applied with caution. There are patients with neurosis or personality disorder who respond not at all to any of these drugs; we would not therefore infer that their egos are strong. The existence of either of these two conditions implies ego weakness, but it is a weakness in a dimension or parameter of ego function different from those just described. We must also remember that, while susceptibility to drug-induced regression indicates ego weakness, immunity to it may not necessarily reflect ego strength but perhaps physiologic resistance to the chemical influence of the drug.

When the abrupt and uncontrolled regression occasionally witnessed in psychoanalytic practice can be controlled with drug therapy, we can observe in "slow motion" the patient's struggle with external stress. For example, when we first see a depressed or psychotic patient, we attempt to guess from the information obtained what the precipitating stress might have been. When the patient recovers from his illness without the help of organic measures, he often turns away from the troublesome situation and attempts to maintain his recovery by denial. If the therapist attempts to confront the patient with the conflict that he sees, he will encounter vigorous resistance. When the patient recovers with the help of chemical agents, he is frequently more courageous in facing pathogenic stress and it becomes easier to help him to deal with these stresses. I resume our discussion of the second case study.

> When I first saw the patient and talked with her husband, I guessed that, although her personality disorder dated back to childhood, the precipitating cause of her breakdown was her husband's need to tightly control every aspect of her life. In her depressive position, she denied resentment against him, and in her "high" state she refused to confront the issue. However, after she had been stabilized by a carefully titrated formula combining both tranquilizer and antidepression medication, she began slowly and deliberately to resume her struggle against him, the struggle in which her psychotic acting out had originated previously. Now, however, she had the courage to pursue a moderate, reasonable course and, with my encouragement, to withstand her husband's pressure. Even with these chemical and psychotherapeutic supports, when her husband actively resisted her, either with an overt display of anger or with sulking, she regressed briefly for a day or so, expressed guilt, and speculated about death. Nevertheless, gradual progress was made toward working out a more acceptable family dynamic.

Observing, with the psychoanalytic instrument, the process of recovery from depression—a process which with the conventional antidepression agents requires three to four weeks—one sees clearly the complementary weakening of self-directed anger and the overt exhibition of anger against the ambivalently loved object. One finds in almost every case a laboratory-type demonstration of the validity of Freud's proposition that, in melancholic depression, the self-directed hostility is no more than the internalized hostility which had originally been directed against the object.

The schizophrenic patient in remission, confronted with his pathogenic stress, will generate conscious fantasies which are clearly derived from the same unconscious conflicts and fantasied resolutions that gave rise to his delusions. They can now be analyzed at leisure, and the patient can be helped to deal with this stress that had once made him ill.

I come now to perhaps the most controversial of my inferences from my experience with drug therapy: the proposition that, from a psychologic point of view, the parameter of psychic function directly affected by both the tranquilizing and the antidepression agents is psychic energy, more specifically, libidinal energy. I have been trying to promote this theory for twenty-five years; I usually encounter great resistance from analysts and drug therapists alike. The former consider what they refer to pejoratively as the hydraulic model to be obsolete. The latter are impatient with all psychologic theories, being interested primarily in chemical mechanisms and clinical description. I have listened to these objections with due respect, and I have considered alternative theories. Nevertheless, I find that an understanding of what these drugs do can best be described psychologically in terms of increases and decreases in the amounts of libidinal energy available to the ego.

There appears to be sparse mention in the literature about the striking fact that schizophrenia and manic-depressive illness are *both* affected by the same chemical agents. Mania is dissipated by chemical agents that, in susceptible individuals, elicit depression, and depression is dissipated by chemical agents that, in susceptible individuals, elicit mania. One form of schizophrenia (which I call the "high" type) is dissipated by the same chemical agents that dissipate mania and that in susceptible individuals elicit either depression or the "low" type of schizophrenia. The "low" type of schizophrenia is dissipated by chemical agents that dissipate depression and that in susceptible individuals elicit mania or the "high" type of schizophrenia. I infer that the biochemical pathogenesis of both conditions, schizophrenia and manic-depressive illness, is the same—or similar, at least up to the point of psychotic dissociation. Whether the patient response to these changes exhibits the clinical picture of schizophrenia or manic-depressive illness depends upon the constitutional susceptibility of the individual toward ego fracture in the schizophrenic pattern, or simply toward ego inflation or depletion. I believe that what is involved from a metapsychologic point of view is the ego's supply of libido. By changing that with chemical agents, one can in the case of both schizophrenia and manic-depressive illness create, obliterate, or change the clinical picture. In any event, psychoanalytic metapsychology must acknowledge the effects of changes in whatever parameter it is that is influenced by these medications and must find a relation among the several clinical states that are affected by the very same drug.

In summary, I maintain that the action of antidepression drugs can best be described as making libidinal energy available to the ego, which is why, in 1956, Kline and I called them "psychic energizers." The increase in energy for the depressed patient makes it possible for him to recover from depression, and if he is given too much medication, he becomes manic. The schizophrenic patient, given this energy, will become more psychotic. Similarly, I propose that the action of tranquilizing drugs can best be described as making libidinal energy unavailable to the ego; the manic or "high" schizophrenic patient will be brought down to remission, or, in the case of susceptible patients, to depression or to a depressive expression of schizophrenia.

In selecting this theory, or if you prefer, metaphor, I was obviously accepting Freud's psychoenergetic theory; my observations of the effects of these drugs confirm his speculations.

One can ask: is this theory necessary? Is it not sufficient to record and to become familiar with the known actions of these substances? For practical purposes, one can content oneself with becoming familiar with the known actions and using the drugs accordingly. However, if one wishes to squeeze the maximum therapeutic value out of these medications, to use them imaginatively for solving clinical problems, and to understand their influence on the analytic process, it is helpful to work with some theoretical frame of reference. For example, the idea of titrating tranquilizing and energizing drugs together for the treatment of schizophrenic patients with depressive tendencies may seem obvious now, but it was not so obvious two decades ago when I first described this procedure. The idea of trying it was derived directly from the libido hypothesis.

Finally, I should like to present another phenomenon and its accompanying theoretical basis. I have already described what I have called the struggle against depression, which consists of various maneuvers evinced before an individual becomes definitively depressed but after a threat of impending depression is unconsciously perceived. I adduced, as evidence of the relation between these states and depression, the fact that they can be dissipated by the administration of energizing drugs; I proposed that the state of overactivity that I called paradoxic hypermotivation, which includes most instances of hypomania and mania, represents an attempt to cope with impending depression by eliciting an emergency energy supply. When additional libidinal energy is made available by an antidepression drug, the need for the paradoxic hypermotivation subsides, and the mania disappears. This proposed explanation of the clinical observations is actually an application of the libido theory of drug actions which I find so useful. Actually, it is an elaboration or corollary of the basic statements I have offered above. This corollary states that when the ego's supply of libido is somehow threatened, the ego can draw upon an emergency supply, with the result that the patient exhibits a clinically observable overactivity. Making supplementary supplies available, for example, by drug therapy, dissipates the overactivity.

At one point I became interested in some reports that phenothiazine and thioxanthene tranquilizers were useful for the treatment of melancholic depression and concurrent reports by other investigators that they were not. When I tried these substances for this purpose, I quickly learned why the reports conflicted; whether or not the tranquilizer exerts an antidepression effect depends upon the dose administered. I learned that many depressed patients will improve with relatively small doses of these agents, but when a certain low threshold dose is exceeded, the antidepression effect disappears and is replaced by an intensification of the depression. What we have, then, is an inverted U-shaped or J-shaped dose-response curve with respect to antidepression response.

Especially interesting is the fact that we already have the theory to help us understand this phenomenon. A small dose of tranquilizer, not sufficient to induce or aggravate definitive depression, acts to establish a depressive threat. The latter then induces a paradoxical hypermotivation which clinically appears as remission of the depressive state. Above a threshold dose, the tranquilizing agent defeats the defensive mechanism and reinforces the spontaneous depressive tendency.

Theoretically, by titrating carefully the amount of tranquilizing drug, one should be able to establish any of the states of the struggle against depression. Actually, this is difficult, because in many patients the susceptibility to this mechanism is limited and because the fixed dosage forms of medication make minute adjustments impractical.

That this is indeed an appropriate description of what happens and not an ad hoc rationalization of the properties of a single group of chemicals is indicated by the fact that similar phenomena are exhibited by chemically different but pharmacologically similar agents.

When a patient has been protected against depression by an antidepression agent, and that agent is then withdrawn, in many instances the first response to withdrawal will be a paradoxic hypermotivation, often with some euphoria. Depressive collapse follows only after the brief appearance of one or more of the variants of the struggle against depression we have been considering.

A few patients respond to tricyclic antidepression therapy within a day or two with elevation of mood and increased activity, sometimes with surprisingly small doses. I infer that in these instances the tricyclic antidepresssion agent, by virtue of its similarity to a phenothiazine, acts as a weak tranquilizer and therefore can elicit a paradoxic hypermotivation.

If a patient is given an antidepression drug in a dose too low to relieve depression, the addition of a small amount of tranquilizing agent will often elicit clinical relief from depression—actually a paradoxical hypermotivation. The antidepression response is stronger than that which the tranquilizer could elicit when given alone, and the patient will tolerate a higher dose of the tranquilizer, without becoming more depressed, than he could tolerate without the antidepression or energizing drug. The subthreshold dose of energizer primes the hypermotivation mechanism, and the small dose of tranquilizer activates it. With this technique it becomes possible to achieve not only relief from depression but to aim at a specific phase of the struggle against depression, for example, to choose between paradoxic hypermotivation and dependent clinging, or perhaps to choose some intermediate state.

We have here, then, a simple but reasonable elaboration of libido theory, consistent with Freud's metapsychology, congenial to the mode of operation of the central nervous system (that is, responding with activation to a small degree of irritation and with reduction in activity when the irritation becomes greater), and useful for the sophisticated practice of drug therapy.

Drug therapy can be regarded as a threat to psychoanalysis by psychoanalysts only if a narrow view of psychoanalysis is taken. If we attempt to explore the ways in which drug therapy can be coordinated with psychoanalysis in both practice and theory, I believe that we shall find that these two subdisciplines of psychiatry complement and enrich each other.

In practice, the availability of drug therapy augments the resources of the analyst for dealing with patients who become depressed or psychotic during the course of treatment and for accepting for treatment such patients in a state of illness. I am not persuaded that there is as much to be gained by emphasizing the problems created by the combined treatment as there is by emphasizing its advantages.

The observations that become available as a result of drug treatment deserve the interest of every conscientious psychiatrist and psychoanalyst. They draw attention to clinical states not previously recognized. They establish and delineate connections between clinical states hitherto only vaguely appreciated. They permit distinctions between clinical states hitherto undifferentiated. For example, the phobia serving the clinging need of the struggle against depression will respond to antidepression drug treatment, while the phobia of neurosis will not. From the point of view of psychoanalytic theory, we learn from drug therapy how to distinguish the fixed characteristics of the personality from the reversible characteristics imposed by the illness, the details of the processes of pathogenesis and recovery, how to estimate one component of ego strength, and new respect for Freud's speculations about libido theory.

It is ironic, perhaps, that no psychiatrist is in as advantageous a position to study drug therapy as the analyst; no other psychiatrist has the opportunity to watch the psychic processes so carefully and for so long. Therefore, the psychoanalyst will be able to understand with special clarity the psychologic workings of these substances and how they can best be used for the benefit of the patient.

CHAPTER 7

The Relationship of Psychopharmacology and Schizophrenia

Otto Allen Will, Jr.

IT IS NOT EASY to define in generally acceptable terms exactly what is meant by "schizophrenia." Every definition somehow seems to be inadequate. The late Lawrence Kubie referred to the concept of schizophrenia as "this combination of a misconception and a misnomer [that] has misled us up a blind alley" (Kubie, 1969). Thomas Szasz writes: "There is, in short, no such thing as schizophrenia. Schizophrenia is not a disease, but only the name of an alleged disease" (Szasz, 1976).

However defined, and whether or not extant, behaviors that are labeled schizophrenia are common, troublesome, and require response. They are certainly not easily, or properly, ignored. Moreover, they constitute a major human difficulty of personal, social, and economic significance. In 1975 Gunderson and Mosher wrote: "The cost of schizophrenia has been estimated at 11.6 to 19.5 billion dollars annually. About two-thirds of this cost is due to lack of productivity by schizophrenic patients and about one-fifth to treatment costs. . . . The cost in human suffering to those with schizophrenia is inestimable."

In a general operational sense the following may be said about schizophrenic behavior:

1. It is a condition of the human being and is closely related to the human's symbolizing ability.
2. It is a state in which there is a strong attachment to other people and great distrust and fear of such attachment.
3. In an effort to maintain some semblance of the vitally needed human relationship, there are developed profound distortions of communication that interfere with understanding and contribute to the sense of personal strangeness, resentment, and despair.
4. There is a reduction in the ability to control the contents of awareness, leading to the feeling of madness accompanied by such phenomena as hallucinations, nightmares, misperceptions and pseudo-explanatory delusions, and the terrifying sensation of disorganization and "falling into pieces."
5. There is felt an urgent need to "do something" about phenomena that seem to have no explanation and that make no sense in terms of the person's own experience.
6. As social and interpersonal relationships are increasingly jeopardized or destroyed by these events, the hope of avoiding being exposed as crazy leads to withdrawal and negativism, further complicating any efforts to increase the human contact that might favor improvement.
7. Whatever identity as a person has been attained is unstable, becomes threatened, and may be lost, adding to the experience of personal and general annihilation.
8. There are revealed long-standing doubts about one's personal value and an isolating and deadly loneliness.

In 1975 Grinker and Holzman wrote the following:

> Pending the outcome of a number of focused laboratory studies, we believe that the following qualities distinguish the young schizophrenic patients from those who are not so diagnosed: (1) the presence of a disorder of thinking, even though it is subtly present; (2) a striking quality of diminished capacity to experience pleasure, particularly in interpersonal relationships; (3) a strong characterological dependence on people; (4) a noteworthy impairment of competence; (5) an exquisitely vulnerable sense of self-regard.
>
> We would suppose that these five qualities reflect a more basic,

hypothetical dysfunction in maintaining the kind of organization necessary for appropriate, adaptive orientation to one's surroundings and to oneself. This basic disorder, we would further hypothesize, need not lead inevitably to psychosis.

It will be evident that the above descriptions are of phenomena that are closely related in varying degrees to the experiences we call normal. That is, they are not entirely foreign to many, if not all of us, in both waking and dreaming states.

In discussing mental health and disorder it is necessary to be aware of conceptual models that may be used. Schizophrenia can be considered in terms of one or more of the following models:

1. The *medical,* in which psychiatric disorders are held to be illnesses or diseases fundamentally much like those usually treated by the physician, with attention given to possible genetic, traumatic, infectious, anatomical, neurophysiological-biochemical difficulties. Treatment is, when possible, directed toward determining and removing the cause and repairing the injury that has resulted, all with a focus on prevention.
2. The *psychologic,* in which the problems reflect vicissitudes and inadequacies of development. Interpersonal intervention is used to facilitate understanding and modification of destructive ways of living.
3. The *behavioral,* in which troublesome behaviors are understood as reflections of learning. Therapy is directed toward the reinforcement of desirable behavior and the extinguishing of that which is considered hurtful.
4. The *social,* in which pathological behaviors are viewed as miniaturized, distorted, or even accurate representations of the social systems in which they have developed and exist.
5. The *existential,* in which the person is considered in terms of the "totality" of his existence with its systems of morality and values, the "illness" being "a way of life."

There are more personal systems, sometimes not clearly recognized or consciously accepted, that constitute a therapist's views of what is right or wrong and "how things ought to be" (Lazare, 1973).

Currently, the emphasis in the field is on the medical model, the value of which is reinforced by studies in genetics, biochemistry, physiology, and pharmacology, by the social pressures to do something for the many in need, and by the economic requirement to demonstrate treatment effectiveness within a traditional medical doctor-patient relationship framework. In my work as a psychotherapist I find each of the models to be informative, but I continue to work largely within the second, or psychologic, model, supported by these others and by studies in comparative animal behavior.

The following comments from articles in the field of ethology are helpful in understanding schizophrenic behavior:

> The ethological approach to understanding behavior is not a simple process that begins with general hypotheses and moves directly to more specific one-to-one causal statements, but rather is one that attempts to account for complexity, usually through progressively specifying a number of behavioral determinants and the conditions that facilitate or inhibit their impact. In short, there are genetic, environmental, physiological, anatomical, and learning components to most behaviors and the understanding of behavior requires that these components be studied simultaneously (McGuire and Fairbanks, 1977).
>
> Disorganization on the individual level is commonly produced by a combination of three situational factors—a high level of motivation, inability to escape from the situation, and inability to adapt to the situation. . . . The first task of diagnosis becomes that of determining which system or systems are involved: social, organismic, physiological, or genetic. If more than one is involved, as is usually the case, it becomes a matter of clinical judgement as to where the most effective remedial action can be taken (Scott, 1977).

A psychotherapist can do nothing about a genetic defect. If such defects exist, they have not been evident in my patients, who have exhibited behavioral changes that appear to me to be a result of a variety of learning experiences. Modification of a hurtfully stressful situation can often be accomplished by moving to a different location or working with the constituents of a social milieu—family, community, or hospital. Psychotherapy, as the term is used here, is concerned with behavioral reorganization, which is sometimes facilitated by the use of drugs to reduce excessive anxiety and disorganization.

Reasons for Treatment

In considering problems of treatment, we must establish the reasons for treatment. The more common reasons are as follows:

1. A person suffers pain, disablement, malfunctioning, and some form of distress from which he wishes to be relieved. Therapeutic efforts are directed toward the alleviation of the distress as the first priority.

2. A major aim of therapy is to bring about cure and to restore a person to a previous state of good health or, in some instances, to a state which is an improvement over that which he has known in the past.

3. The troubled person may not complain or directly seek help, but his behavior may disturb others of the community in which he lives. As this disturbance is felt to be intolerable, efforts will be made to change what the particular person is doing. In brief, he may be advised to seek treatment—or even forced to accept it against his wishes.

4. Treating a person who does not ask for it, and may reject it, raises ethical problems that cannot be dismissed or easily solved. The undesirable behavior is to be eliminated (perhaps through cure), modified, or somehow concealed. If no cure is possible at that time, and modification is not adequate, the suffering person is sent away or eliminated in the service of community needs. Again I quote from the article on ethology by McGuire and Fairbanks (1977):

> It is worth noting that normal-abnormal distinctions appear to be made by nearly all animal and human species thus far studied and that persistent abnormal behavior on the part of a group member leads either to rejection from or direct attack by the group. Thus, the degree to which behavioral labeling is purely cultural in origin and, by inference, eliminatable, must be questioned (p. 11).

There is often a close relationship between control, coercion, and what methods may be identified as treatment. It is necessary, at least, to distinguish between acts taken for the welfare of the person and those taken for the sake of the community. The needs of these two are not always identical, but whenever possible they should not be confused. It is obvious that psychiatric care is intimately involved with this matter.

5. Treatment procedures may be instituted primarily for the help that may be brought to the patient through their use. From them may be derived further understanding of the disordered behavior and the circumstances (personal and environmental) in which it exists. This secondary gain cannot in itself be easily justified as a reason for the treatment, however.

A Cursory Survey of Treatments in Schizophrenia

If a person comes to be known as schizophrenic, it is very likely that he will be introduced to numerous explanations for his difficulty and probably will receive a variety of treatments for it, each more or less related to current concepts of causation. Treatments range from seemingly benign efforts to provide comfortable retreats or asylums in which the troubled person can find a temporary, or even permanent, escape from the pressure of living (including those that demand change or cure at any cost) to intrusive, aggressive, violent attempts to treat that can be cruel. During my own experience in the field I have had direct or indirect contact with the methods of treatment that are listed here.

1. An attitude of nihilism, reflecting the idea that the organism is biologically inadequate, is destined to deteriorate, will show no lasting improvement, and will likely be made worse by any form of intervention.
2. The removal of supposed foci of infection in an effort to eliminate their toxic products that may have brought about the pathological condition.
3. The intrathecal injection of horse serum with the purpose of producing a sterile meningismus.
4. The intravenous injection of gold salts as in the once popular treatment of arthritis.
5. The production of artificial hyperthermia as in the treatment of central nervous system syphilis.
6. The induction of prolonged sleep.
7. The use of insulin to produce coma and sometimes seizures.
8. The use of intravenous Metrazol (pentylenetetrazol) to produce generalized seizures.
9. The application of nitrogen and oxygen to produce seizures.
10. ECT or EST, now referred to as electrically induced seizures.
11. Various forms of psychosurgery.
12. Implantation of bits of metal into the brain, to which bits externally generated electric impulses are directed.
13. Dialysis of the blood.
14. Massive doses of vitamins, sometimes combined with various medications and electroshock.
15. Behavioral conditioning.
16. Various forms of group exercises, such as group therapy, family therapy, milieu therapy, or sociotherapy.
17. Psychotherapy of many types, including ''direct'' psychoanalysis, and so on.
18. Antipsychotic drugs as discussed in this conference by experts in psychopharmacology.

The following comment on schizophrenia by Leo Hollister (1973) reflects a current and influential view of the problem:

> Older notions that schizophrenia is a reaction to social-psychological influences, such as that it represents a disordered learning process initiated and sustained by conflicting messages from mother, have few remaining adherents. The present tendency is to regard schizophrenia as a genetically determined disorder with biological mechanisms whose phenotypic expression may be influenced in part by life experiences. . . . The term "antipsychotic" drug should in no way imply that these drugs are curative. . . . They may simply relieve secondary symptoms of schizophrenia and arrest or ameliorate the natural course of the disorder (p. 13).
>
> The ideal psychotherapeutic drug would: (a) cure or alleviate the pathogenic mechanisms of the symptom or disorder; (b) be rapidly effective; (c) be nonhabituating and lack potential for creating dependence; (d) benefit most or all patients for whom it is indicated; (e) not have tolerance develop; (f) have minimum toxicity on the therapeutic range; (g) have a low incidence of secondary side effects; (h) would not be lethal in overdoses; (i) be adaptable both to inpatients and outpatients; and (j) not impair any cognitive, perceptual, or motor functions. No such drug exists, but to a fairly surprising degree many of the available drugs meet the majority of these desiderata (p. 12).

The Choice of the Form of Treatment

The choice of a particular form of treatment is dependent upon several factors, singly or in combination. As an example, consider the problem of choice confronted by the parents of a twenty-year-old son who experienced an acute psychotic episode at the age of eighteen and had been in some form of psychiatric program since that time. I list a few of the elements that contributed to their decisions about therapy. It is important to note that the son did not wish to participate in any therapeutic program.

1. The parents' concept of the difficulty, schizophrenia in this case, is a major factor in the selection of a course of action. The parents of this boy were afraid that the illness was in some way genetic and could thus never be cured in the sense that the young man could some day lead a life considered to be productive by conventional standards. The mother expressed concern about being what was called at one time (unfortunately) "schizophrenogenic": she puzzled about what she must have done "wrong" in raising three children, the second of whom was the patient and the others "normal." Both parents were ashamed, felt

somehow disgraced, and expressed a feeling of abhorrence about the son's behavior. The father seemed to be more secure if the difficulties were said to be a disease "like any other, only we don't know what causes it or what to do." In the course of the discussion, they spoke of their love for their child and also of their feelings of frustration, discouragement, and anger. They wished that the trouble would go away—and hesitantly realized that they might wish that *he* would go away. "Sometimes I think he'd be better off dead," said the father. "Only if it were God's will," added the mother, who then said, "If I were superstitious I'd say we'd been cursed." Being modern, well-educated people, they turned to medicine and what they knew as the scientific approach.

2. Selection also depends on the one who gives advice about what to do. In this case, the decision for care was made by police officers who took the young man into custody when he caused a disturbance by shouting obscenities and disrobing in public. He was taken to a hospital and given medicine intramuscularly despite his protests. A consultant then described the patient's difficulties as a disease process that could be held in check through the use of medication but could not thereby be cured. The next year passed with some improvement at times but with recurrent relapses and rehospitalization. Attention was then turned to megavitamin therapy with the addition of lithium, and marked improvement followed. As he improved, however, the patient left the hospital and terminated therapy with a subsequent return to a condition of near-apathy and a marginal, lonely existence.

3. In this state of withdrawal and "refusal to accept help" the young man was once again on the way to becoming a public nuisance. He was remanded to the local state hospital, from which he was rapidly discharged to a program of community care which he soon left.

4. The parents then sought advice about a program of more prolonged intensive psychotherapy in a hospital. The cost of such treatment was, to them, prohibitive, and there was no guarantee of its success.

The response that is given to a patient is thus dependent upon the motivation of the patient, the beliefs of the family members, the concepts of disease and treatment currently popular or known in the community, the authority who recommends a particular course of action, the public disturbance caused by the patient's behavior, the local tolerance of that behavior, the facilities available for treatment, the costs involved, and the funds (insurance, public, or private) that can be drawn upon for payment.

The Situation as a Determinant of Treatment

When the situation is not perceived as immediately critical (such as during wartime or civilian disasters which require immediate crisis intervention) there are many influences that determine the form of treatment that will be provided for people suffering from disturbances labeled as psychiatric. Among these are the amount of public and private financial support that is available. There is, obviously, much competition for the use of these funds and many more-or-less persuasive arguments for the support of one enterprise rather than another. Good advertising is required to sell the product to the buyer—private corporation, local, state, or federal government, or the taxpayer who is a major contributor to any decision regarding the use of money.

In determining the allocation of economic and social support, certain practical questions which are not always clearly recognized or stated openly may arise. For example: Which group has the greatest need? Which contributes "most" to the "good" of society—if the terms "most" and "good" can be defined in any generally satisfactory way? Which has the greater political strength and the better program of advertising or public relations? And which group is considered to be more worthy of helping, treating, or saving?

These questions are not pleasant, and there are no quick or easy answers to them, despite the various solutions, both simplistic and complex, that have been proposed. We cannot avoid being confronted with a consideration of the extent and limitation of resources and of their use and distribution. We do not always ask some of these questions openly, but through our public and private actions we do give answers to them, often covertly and with accompanying denial of what we do.

In our society there are groups of people who are not highly regarded, despite some rhetoric to the contrary. In brief, we don't like them (with individual exceptions); we feel uncomfortable or guilty when we are told (and guess, or know) that we play some part in their creation and continuance; we don't know what to do about them or our feelings about them; and we wish that they would (for the most part) disappear or go away without the necessity of our recognizing the wish to eliminate or destroy them. Reference here is to (a) the poor, (b) the criminal, (c) the aged, (d) certain troublesome adolescents, (e) outsiders (people felt to be intolerably different from us), (f) the mentally defective (however defined), and (g) psychiatric patients, particularly those who are psychotic and require long-term care.

Another influencing factor may be the rapid increase of population in the country, the migratory characteristics of our life, and an accompanying decrease of feelings of acquaintance, relatedness, and responsibility for the other person. Without direct personal contact, usually over weeks or months, it is easy to come to feel that all people are strangers. Again, knowledge of such matters is beyond the range of my professional competence.

A factor which may hinder us in recognizing clearly the reality and seriousness of these influences in determining the form of treatment or intervention is the wish to find some cheap and quick, almost magical, solution for these troublesome behaviors. We know that a major—if not *the* major—cost of treatment is in personnel. The use of human beings as therapeutic agents is expensive, and it is understandable that we look for more effective and cheaper agents whose actions are more predictable.

We would also prefer an agent which is safe, effective, and so readily available and low in cost that it could be given to any person who needed it.

Today, we in psychiatry should recognize the functioning of the concept of triage, defined in the OED as "The act of sorting according to quality." The more socially sophisticated forms of therapy, usually involving the interaction of a variety of professional skills, are not usually available to those who can't pay their way. This is not, of course, simply a decision to treat those people who have the best prognosis or who are most likely (if we can judge) to contribute to society's betterment.

The Current Scene

In discussing the selection of a mode of treatment for the psychotic schizophrenic patient, it is useful to consider current trends that influence such a determination. I select a few of these as they operate in areas of the nation with which I am somewhat familiar.

1. The state hospitals have for many years been described as "warehouses," unfit places for the administration of adequate treatment. They have been poorly supported financially, and the morale of patients and staff members is generally poor. No longer are these institutions considered to be "retreats," "asylums," or refuges in the better sense of these words. In order to gain admission, a prospective patient may be required to wait several weeks. The length of stay is usually not long, as treatment is directed toward rapid discharge.

2. The state hospital patient is designated to be returned to his community, but he can be assured of no acceptance there. Without private funds, he is likely to be on some form of relief through public aid and may lead a marginal existence in poor housing conditions.

3. It is not likely that the discharged patient will be welcomed back into his family, even if he has a family that could provide shelter. The halfway house is a useful part of a rehabilitation program, but these are not easily established or maintained. Much persuasion is required for people to accept such an institution in their community; they are afraid. They will say such things as: "Property values will fall. Those people (patients) are dangerous; it's not good for the children to be near them. They will act crazy and our friends won't come here any more. They'd be happier somewhere out in the country—away from the town." I have seen community meetings about these questions come close to violence.

The halfway house may accommodate only eight to ten patients, and many houses are required to provide adequate space for those eligible. As the push to discharge patients increases, more disturbed people are pushed into these houses, causing a concomitant increase in violence. Patients who are unable to adjust to the requirements of living in these facilities are discharged to the street or are returned to the state hospital, which usually sends them back in short order. The police frequently act as intermediaries between the state and local agencies.

4. Although we speak of rehabilitation, many of these discharged patients are simply being maintained outside of hospitals in states of chronicity. There is a need for a system of day-care centers, clinics for ambulatory patients, activities programs, education and job training, and psychiatric supervision of the use of medication and of overall care. From what I have observed, the support for all of this is minimal.

5. Many psychiatric units in general hospitals provide treatment for only a few days—for a five-day critical period, for example. Treatment in such units consists largely of reducing the severity of the outward manifestations of disorder and preparing the patient to go elsewhere. There often is no clearly defined or satisfactory "elsewhere."

6. Without counseling, supervision, and some form of psycho-therapy, the patient may drop out of a program, give up whatever treatment has been provided, and wander about until he comes to public attention once again through suicide, death by other means, physical illness, or obvious socially or personally intolerable craziness.

7. Over thirty years ago, in one of the then wealthiest counties in the United States, there were no facilities for the emergency housing of

the acutely disturbed—suicidal and psychotic people. They were often placed in the local jail, where some remained for several months. Today, in one of the large cities the same condition exists, although the length of stay may be shorter.

What do these phenomena have to do with the use of medication with the schizophrenic patient? It is difficult to discuss treatment procedures without attending to the situations in which that treatment is to be given and to the goals which are supposed to be achieved. I think that we—the public and the profession—often ask too much from any new trend in therapy; we want the "answer," we ask that the problem be solved quickly and economically so that we can get on with other business which is more agreeable or seemingly more profitable to us. When the problem isn't solved, we are disappointed, feel betrayed, find our faith diminishing, and may accept the appealing idea that the patients are hopeless and the professionals are fools. There is a great temptation to seek a miracle drug, some equivalent of what was called, in days past, Ehrlich's "magic bullet."

The antipsychotic drugs have been demonstrated to be of great value in the modification of a number of dangerously crippling disturbances, but I do not think that the results of their use are just those often depicted in the journal advertisements that come to my attention. There are the "before and after" pictures of the disturbed person; there is the previously deeply troubled patient who, with the help of some drug, is now happily and efficiently working at a job or talking (apparently pleasantly) with the benign and respected physician. This is not the life of therapy with schizophrenic patients as I have known it. They usually manage to come to see me, but I am more often treated like a sparring partner and am annointed more with anger and doubt than with friendly appreciation.

Because of the magnitude of the psychiatric problems and their associated factors, some of which have been mentioned in the foregoing, there is great pressure to use medications more for the control of behavior rather than as an important adjunct to more comprehensive treatment. I think that it is proper to control behavior with medication, for example, when the welfare of the patient and his surroundings are seriously threatened by what he does. I do not favor the substitution of medication, or other restraint, for the human relationships which are of fundamental importance in building a trusting and healing attitude toward oneself and other people. If the use of medication comes to be accepted only, or primarily, as a means of control, its truly valuable functions may be minimized or disregarded. I refer to such functions as the reduction of anxiety and disorganization to the end that the patient is enabled to cooperate with procedures designed to promote more enduring personality change.

Other Problems

The prescribing and administration of antipsychotic medications to patients is no longer as simple a procedure as once it may have seemed to be. The following is a quotation from the *San Francisco Chronicle* of March 12, 1980.

> A federal judge ordered California hospitals and psychiatrists yesterday to obtain informed consent from voluntary mental patients for every "mind altering" drug given to them.
>
> [The] American Civil Liberties attorney . . . who helped bring a 1978 suit to expand the rights of mental patients, called the decision "a significant break through. It is an overdue recognition of the constitutional rights of mental patients." . . . [B]oth private and mental health institutions must tell voluntary patients what mind-altering drugs are proposed for them, what they will do, and what the possible adverse side effects are, and that the patients have the right to refuse the medication.
>
> The order does not apply to patients involuntarily committed to mental care through legal action.

(See also Amarasingham, 1980; Appelbaum and Gutheil, 1980; Ford, 1980; and Reiser, 1980.)

The proposed consent form that the patient might be asked to sign is impressive; that is, any cautious, not fully trusting person would hesitate to sign it. I shall not attempt to discuss this matter here, but we shall hear much more about it. There is involved not only the question of trust between therapist and patient but also that of the pressure on the profession to act on occasion beyond the functions of healing.

Personal Views

As may be evident, I do not feel fully at ease in making the preceding remarks. I know that the usefulness of psychotherapy, particularly with schizophrenic people, is questioned—but then, it always has been questioned. I myself often feel old-fashioned, if not outmoded, passed by in the rush of current discoveries and theories. In a sense that is true, and I have no complaints. I can only state my views and work to keep myself open to the worthy new concepts that arise.

The schizophrenic people with whom I have worked have reached adolescence without having fallen by the wayside. That is, they did not become marasmic, autistic, or openly schizophrenic before the age of puberty. They have been at least normally intelligent, and their physical needs have been met adequately. They have failed to meet the major tasks of adolescence—developing of intimate relationships, patterning of sexual behavior in a satisfactory fashion, separation from home, further organizing a stable identity, and so on. They have withdrawn in shame and loneliness, attempted suicide, or become acutely or gradually psychotic. They have become engaged in a more-or-less evident struggle for survival that required resolution. Some have died by suicide or misadventure. Others further hid their conflicts through dissociation and became more cautious in engaging in human relationships; they did not welcome the therapeutic approach. Those who developed the hebephrenic or paranoid solution were so walled off that I found it extremely difficult to be of use to them. A few seemed to improve without known official aid and were able to act profitably with their lives. Others continued in their unhappy struggle; as long as they were fighting and had not resorted to the simplified answer, they were approachable and could become accepting—slowly, and with doubt and mistrust—of my presence.

I know that there is nothing "magical" in my own work as a therapist. No patient has, to my knowledge, found me to be empathic, warm, understanding, or very knowledgeable about his/her personal brand of trouble. I am not pleased by these facts, but there is no need for me as a therapist to be pleased with myself. I know that, if I continue to be present, bonds will be established between me and the patient, and I believe that these can often be put to good use. The establishment of such bonds or ties is based on biological fact; I don't have to do anything extraordinary in bringing this about. Of course, I must be there and prevent harm to the patient, myself, or others. I try to help the patient to become a good teacher to me. In a general way, I know something about the patient, but in a more personal and particular way I am ignorant. To be a good teacher, the patient must know his subject well—what he experiences, who he is, how he views his world, how he behaves, how others view him, and so on. It is his job to teach me about these matters, and in doing that I think that his living will improve. As a student I must be curious and have the desire to learn. If I act like a know-it-all, or like someone who doesn't need to learn and can somehow read minds, the patient-teacher may lose interest in the work and become discouraged with the arduous task of educating a therapist who never seems to understand or grasp the essentials of what goes on.

Of course, we work closely with other staff members. We do our best to help the patient's relatives comprehend what we are about, knowing that change in relationships and personality, although desired, can be painful and at times disastrous. We don't want anyone to become damaged in this process. We seek growing attachment, trust, self revelation, and confidence—and the strength to deal with the inevitable separation.

I do not turn to medication as the first resort. I am asking the patient to reveal himself as he is, and I don't want to interfere immediately with his response by chemical or other means. I do use medication if the patient's behavior is seriously threatening to anyone, but I don't do this "automatically." First I try to see what we human beings can do with our presence.

It is evident that I have not had the experience of maintaining patients on medication. Also, it should be noted, I do not advocate continuing indefinitely in a deteriorating interpersonal situation or in one in which there is no detectable evidence of increasing trust and clarity. In such a case we may use medication or other resources—the transfer to another therapist, for example.

I do not think that every patient can be treated in just the same way—or should be. I also do not think that schizophrenia will be eradicated through any of our efforts; we must work at becoming more effective in giving help to those people who are afflicted. It is important that we do not abandon ourselves to the despair of our patients, although they often seem to invite us to do so. They are not hopeless, even though some may show little change through our efforts. They are much more like "us" (whoever we are) than they are different.

I do recommend that some of the intensive individualized psychotherapeutic work with schizophrenic people be continued; the longitudinal study of personality is not a rapid or easy source of results, but it is, in my view, a useful way to learn more about ourselves as well as to help our patients.

References

Amarasingham, L. R. Social and cultural perspectives on medication refusal. *Amer. J. Psychiat. 137:*3 (March, 1980) 353–358, 1980.

Appelbaum, P. A., and Gutheil, T. G. Drug refusal: A study of psychiatric inpatients. *Amer. J. Psychiat. 137:*3 (March, 1980) 340–346, 1980.

FORD, M. DEG. The psychiatrist's double bind: The right to refuse medication. *Amer. J. Psychiat. 137:*3 (March, 1980) 332–339, 1980.

GRINKER, R. R. and HOLZMAN, P. S. Schizophrenic pathology in young adults: A clinical study. *Arch. Gen. Psycho. 28:*2 (February, 1973) 168–175, 1973.

GUNDERSON, J. G., and MOSHER, L. The cost of schizophrenia. *Amer. J. Psychiat. 132:*901–6 (1975).

HOLLISTER, L. E. *Clinical use of psychotherapeutic drugs.* Springfield, Ill: Charles C Thomas, 1973; pp. 12–13.

KUBIE, L. S. Multiple fallacies in the concept of schizophrenia: Problems of psychosis. Excerpta Medica International Congress Series, No. 194, Proceedings of the International Colloquium on Psychosis, Montreal, November 5–8, 1969, pp. 301–311.

LAZARE, A. Hidden conceptual models in clinical psychiatry. *New Eng. J. Med. 288:*7 345–51; 1973.

MCGUIRE, M. T., and FAIRBANKS, L. A. Ethology: Psychiatry's bridge to behavior. In McGuire, M. T., and Fairbanks, L. A. (Eds.), *Ethological psychiatry: Psychopathology in the context of evolutionary biology.* New York, San Francisco, and London: Grune and Stratton, 1977; pp. 1–40.

REISER, S. J. Refusing treatment for mental illness: Historical and ethical dimensions. *Amer. J. Psychiat. 137:*3 329–331, 1980.

SCOTT, J. P. Agonistic behavior: Adaptive and maladaptive organization. In McGuire, M. T., and Fairbanks, L.A. (Eds.), *Ethological psychiatry: Psychopathology in the context of evolutionary biology.* New York, San Francisco, and London: Grune and Stratton, 1977; pp. 193–209.

SZASZ, T. *Schizophrenia: The sacred symbol of psychiatry.* New York: Basic Books, Inc., 1976, p. 191.

CHAPTER 8

The Interaction of Drug Therapy and Family Treatment in Schizophrenia

Michael J. Goldstein and
Eliot H. Rodnick

DURING THE LAST FEW YEARS, the community mental health center movement at the national and local levels has generated a treatment model for acute schizophrenia composed of two phases—a brief inpatient phase, measured in days, followed by an extended period of aftercare in the community. In the old system, relatively complete remission of schizophrenic symptoms was the goal; in this new system of inpatient treatment, minimal remission of only the most acute and disorganizing symptoms is the goal. It is believed that the balance of the recovery process can be more effectively achieved once the patient has been returned to community life.

While this new model emphasizes aftercare in the community, it has been far from certain what this means, particularly for the acute, young, first-admission schizophrenic. A number of key questions concerning effective modes of treatment in community settings still remain to be answered. First, what role should antipsychotic drugs play in the aftercare program? We know well the impact and significance of these drugs during extended inpatient treatment of schizophrenics (May,

1968). But given our knowledge of the difficulties involved in continued acceptance by patients of these drugs following discharge, how can they be utilized in community-based treatment of acute schizophrenics and for how long?

Second, many patients released from community mental health centers still manifest residual symptoms and adjustment difficulties. What models of social therapies are appropriate to deal with the reintegration of such patients into the community and perhaps to prevent future psychotic breakdowns? The issue of psychotherapeutic approaches to schizophrenia has moved to a new arena and deals with a different stage of the illness. No longer do we ask whether psychotherapy is effective in aiding the patient to reconstitute from psychotic confusion. Now we ask whether, once some partial restitution has been effected, social therapies can play a significant role in the treatment of schizophrenia (May, 1976, and Schooler, 1978). Can the interacting roles of drugs and social therapies be utilized to maximize the effects of each? The research project described herein represents one attempt to attend to these issues.

Method

Design of Study

The study, conducted with my colleagues Eliot Rodnick and Phillip May, was carried out at the Ventura Mental Health Center in California. In this center, schizophrenic patients are released to the community after an average of fourteen days hospitalization. A previous study (Evans, Goldstein, and Rodnick, 1973) on a sample of all consecutive schizophrenic admissions over an eighteen-month period in that center found that 45 percent were readmitted for substantial periods within six months of discharge. Further, the majority of readmissions (31 percent) occurred within three to four weeks. Two other facts were noted: First, patients simply did not take the oral dose of phenothiazines prescribed on discharge; second, they rarely used the outpatient supportive social therapy that was provided. Therefore, we developed an experimental design that focused on the first six weeks after discharge (a critical period, according to the above data) and then studied the relative significance of depot phenothiazine treatment and crisis-oriented family therapy carried out during that critical period.

This study involved almost all first-admission schizophrenics in a county of one-half million people. The 2 × 2 factorial design of the study had two levels of maintenance phenothiazine, high and low dosage, and two social therapy conditions, present or absent.

Selection of Patients

All consecutive first and second inpatient admissions to the Ventura Mental Health Center were screened for the presence of schizophrenic symptoms. Independently interviewed by the project psychiatrist and psychologist, each patient was rated on a five-point scale on the probability that he might be schizophrenic (Mosher, Pollin, and Stabenau, 1971). Each patient who passed this initial screening was studied for another two to three days and then rated on the New Haven Schizophrenia Index (Astrachen, Harrow, Adler, et al. 1972). Those who received a score of four or higher (a cutting score found by Astrachan et al. to correlate highly with a clinical diagnosis of schizophrenia) were entered into the study. Of the 104 patients selected for the study, 69 percent were first lifetime admissions, and the balance recent second admissions (during the same calendar year.) They were young (mean age 23.36 years; SD, 4.21) and predominantly white (79 percent), with 14 percent of Hispanic origin and 7 percent black. Forty percent had not graduated from high school, 35 percent were high school graduates, and 25 percent had had some college. Sixty-two percent were single, 15 percent previously married, and 23 percent currently married. They were hospitalized only briefly (mean 14.24 days; SD, 5.97) before discharge to the aftercare program.

After a patient was selected, he and a relative were interviewed separately and informed of the nature of the study. Consent was required from both the patient and the relative for the patient to participate. The patient was informed that he could withdraw from the study at any time.

The Phenothiazine Drug Condition

It was decided to compare a relatively high therapeutic dose level of phenothiazine with a therapeutically marginal or lower dosage of the same drug. The original intent was to use orally administered phenothiazines, but this was not feasible because of a low rate of compliance. Accordingly, we shifted to a longer acting injectable phenothiazine, fluphenazine (Prolixin) enanthate, which successfully solved the problem of medication delivery.

Fluphenazine therapy was started within a day after the patients had been admitted to the center. A test dose of 0.25 ml was given; if no sensitivity was noted, the patient was then assigned by a random method to one of two conditions: high or low dose. Originally we had intended that the high dose should be 1.5 ml and the low dose 0.5 ml, but pilot data suggested that the side effects of the higher dose were too severe. Dosages were therefore reduced in the actual experiment to 1 ml for the high-dose condition and 0.25 ml for the low-dose condition and were kept fixed throughout the study. [While we use the term high dose for the 1-ml condition, it is clear that, in contrast to other studies using this same drug with acute schizophrenic patients (Chien and Cole, 1973), a more appropriate term would be moderate dose.] Prophylactic antiparkinsonian medication was provided routinely: benztropine mesylate, 2 mg intramuscularly with each injection of fluphenazine, and trihexyphenidyl, 5 mg/day orally during both the inpatient and aftercare phases of the study. The study period was typically one to two weeks as an inpatient and a six-week aftercare period as an outpatient. During the inpatient period, if the treating psychiatrist thought that more medication was needed, he was permitted to administer phenothiazine orally. During the aftercare period, three injections were administered at fourteen-day intervals, the first on the day of discharge. The study was single blind, as the patient was blind to dose level but the treating psychiatrist was not. However, all ratings of clinical behavior were carried out by raters blind to drug and family therapy status.

Crisis-Oriented Family Therapy

The social therapy used was family oriented. Here, our original desires or goals were modified by experience. It was our hope, based on other work, that we could move into some kind of relationally oriented family therapy. However, it became obvious that this was not feasible for such disorganized patients. Instead, a crisis-oriented six-session family therapy was devised, directed at the following sequence of objectives:

1. The patient and his family are able to accept the fact that he has had a psychosis.

2. They are willing to identify some of the probable precipitating stresses in his life at the time the psychosis occurred.
3. They attempt to generalize identification of future stresses to which the patient and his family are likely to be vulnerable.
4. They attempt to do some planning on how to minimize or avoid these future stresses.

We find that this concrete form of family therapy can be meaningfully carried out with schizophrenics and their families during this phase of treatment. The primary goal in this therapy is to help the patient and significant others to use the events of the psychosis rather than deflecting attention away from the psychotic episode.

Results

Deliverability and Compliance

Of the 104 patients who agreed to participate in the program, eight withdrew after release from the hospital. Three of these left the area immediately; five remained in the area but rejected compliance with their assigned treatment program. Thus, 92 percent participated in the aftercare program. The treatment refusers came from three groups: high-dose/therapy (two), low-dose/therapy (three), and low-dose/no-therapy (three).

Figure 8–1 presents the rate of relapse within each treatment condition at the end of the six-week controlled trial and at the time of the six-month follow-up contact. During the six-week controlled treatment period, ten patients deteriorated clinically to such an extent that either they had to be rehospitalized or their medication had to be altered substantially—a relapse rate for treatment accepters of 10.4 percent. This is substantially less than the 31 percent rate for the comparable six-week post-discharge period found for a similar consecutive admission study at this same facility (Evans et al., 1973). Relapse diagnoses were ordinarily not the decision of the research team, as they usually involved action by the center's emergency psychiatric team carried out independently of the project team. In cases where the decision to rehospitalize was made by the research staff, a consensus of staff—both blind and nonblind to treatment status—was necessary.

While this is a small number of relapses in which to seek differential trends across treatment conditions or patients' attributes, some suggestive findings do appear. These data indicate that there are two ex-

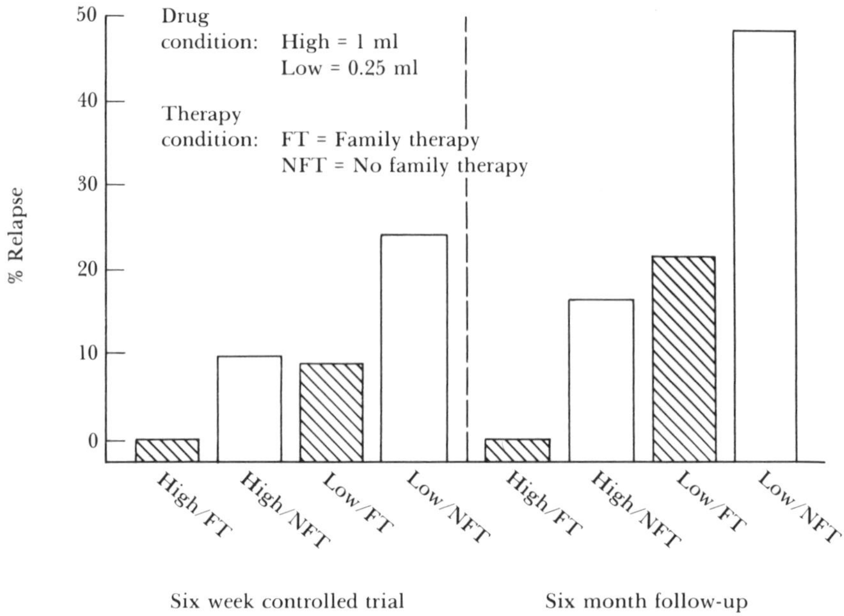

Figure 8–1. Relapse rate within each treatment condition at the end of the six-week controlled trial and at the time of the six month follow-up contact.

tremes in the groups of the sample, the high-dose therapy group with not a single relapse and the low-dose/no-therapy group with 24 percent relapse. The other two conditions fell between these two and do not differ significantly. Only the extremely polarized groups differ at a statistically significant level. The trends in the marginal totals for dose level and therapy effects, while suggestive, are not statistically significant for either factor. Thus, despite the small number of relapsing patients, they are concentrated largely in the group with minimal medication and an absence of family-oriented intervention.

The number of breakdowns following the completion of the controlled period parallels the pattern for the first six weeks. There was not a single relapse in the high-dose/therapy group, while by the six-month point nearly fifty percent of the low-dose/no-therapy group had had some sort of clinical regression. The groupings under the other two conditions had more breakdowns than did the high-dose/therapy group but less than did the low-dose/no-therapy group. Thus, even though the high-dose/therapy patients were no longer receiving therapy and were no longer rigorously assigned to a maintenance medication condition, they continued to remain free of hospitalization for a six-month period.

If we add together the relapses during the controlled period with those that followed into an overall cumulative six-month relapse figure, a significant drug effect ($p < .01$) and a near significant therapy effect ($p < .10$) are found.

Symptomatic Status at End of Aftercare Period

Patients were rated four times (at admission, at discharge, at six weeks, and at six-month follow-up), using the Brief Psychiatric Rating Scale (BPRS) (Overall and Gorham, 1962). The rater was a research psychologist who remained blind to drug and therapy status throughout the six-month period. Factor analysis of admission BPRS ratings was carried out to reduce the 16 scales to a smaller set of dimensions. Fourteen of the scales loaded on four factors, anxious-depression, hostility, emotional withdrawal, and schizophrenic thought. Data were analyzed in two ways, with relapsed patients deleted (all completers), and with last contact ratings used to include all starters in the sample.

Family Therapy Effects

The strongest effects are noted when the endpoint ratings for the relapsers are included in the analysis. Significant effects were found for the family therapy variable on: total BPRS score ($p < .01$); withdrawal ($p < .02$); and anxious depression ($p < .05$), for all patients who began the therapy (all starters). In all instances there was evidence of less residual psychopathology in the samples that received family therapy.

The magnitude of the therapy effect on withdrawal is as significant for all completers as for all starters. Therefore, the impact of the family therapy on withdrawal applies to all cases in the sample. The mean scores on the withdrawal factor are presented separately below for all starters and all completers.

All starters ($p < .02$)		*All completers* ($p < .03$)	
Therapy	No Therapy	Therapy	No Therapy
2.41	3.65	2.39	3.72

If we examine, for the completers, the individual BPRS scales constituting the withdrawal factor, one particularly stands out; *blunted affect* ($p < .005$), in which the therapy cases manifested significantly less flattening of affect at six weeks than did the no-therapy cases.

Analysis of BPRS data at the time of six-month follow-ups was only significant for the withdrawal factor and only so in the group that originally received the high phenothiazine dose. As before, family therapy cases on high dosage showed less residual psychopathology than did comparable no-therapy cases ($p < .05$). However, the therapy advantage, previously observed with patients on low dosage, was no longer observable at the six-month follow-up. Note that the sustained effect on the high-dose group persisted long after those patients were systematically receiving the drug. It suggests a prophylactic effect of the adequate dose upon the retention of family therapy effects over the more extended time period.

Further Analyses of the Family Therapy Process

Up to this point we have been treating psychotherapeutic intervention as a homogenous process applied equally to all patients. However, we recognize that there is considerable variation in styles of therapy and in the ability of patients and therapists to utilize each other's resources.

An analogy may be drawn to a similar issue in pharmacotherapy when patients are assigned medication but often fail to comply. Thus, it has been necessary for researchers to devise methods to assure delivery or at the very least to monitor compliance. We felt that a comparable index of the deliverability of a psychotherapeutic intervention would permit a more accurate appraisal of its effects as well as greater insight into the process of change.

Previously we indicated that the crisis-oriented therapy had relatively specific objectives. Four specific sequential objectives were designated:

1. Acceptance by patient and family that the patient has had a psychotic episode and consensus concerning the important precipitating stresses at the time the psychosis occurred.
2. Development of strategies to prevent the occurrence of identified stresses and for coping when stress occurs.
3. Evaluation of progress in implementation of prevention and coping strategies.
4. Anticipatory planning to prevent future stresses and to cope with those that arise.

In this study, therapists rated the extent to which the patient and participating family members achieved each of the four objectives.

A graduate student, Charles King, and I (King and Goldstein, 1979) hypothesized that the greater the number of therapy objectives attained, the greater the sustained benefit by patient and significant others.

Measures

Achievement of Objectives in Therapy. At the completion of therapy, therapists rated each patient on a five-point scale regarding the extent to which the patient was successful in achieving each of the four therapy objectives. The scale included descriptions of typical patient achievements for each point on the scale for each objective. For the purposes of analysis, the four objectives were treated as a Guttman Scale, with the assumption that achievement of a given objective implied achievement of all of the lower objectives. A patient was considered to have achieved an objective if he was rated three (moderately successful) or above. The highest objective achieved by each patient became his single score for the achievement of objectives in therapy. These scores range from zero to four, distributed as follows: zero, 20.5 percent; one, 20.5 percent; two, 9 percent; three, 9 percent; four, 41 percent. For some analyses subjects were categorized as "achievers" or "nonachievers" of therapy objectives, employing a median split on the highest objective achieved. Thus, subjects who achieved objectives three or four were classified as achievers; those who achieved no higher than objective two are referred to as nonachievers.

Achievers and nonachievers did not differ significantly on the demographic variables of age, marital status, race, education, or father's education. In addition, there was no significant difference between achiever groups in the number of family members participating in therapy sessions.

Ratings of Achievement of Therapy Objectives as a Dependent Variable. First, we examined whether factors observed prior to the initiation of the aftercare family therapy could predict therapists' perceptions of the level of objectives achieved. The variables used were the individual differences measures of sex, premorbid status, paranoid status, GAS (Endicott, Spitzer, Fleiss, et al., 1976) level ratings at admission, and BPRS factor scores at admission and discharge. For the quantitative variables, a median split was used to subdivide groups. In addition, we examined whether assigned drug level (high versus low) was associated with greater success in delivering the therapy model.

None of the individual differences variables or drug levels were found related to therapist ratings of patients' achievement of objectives in therapy.

Next, interactions between individual differences variables and drug levels were examined to determine whether the combination of certain patient attributes and assigned drug levels could predict the therapists' perceived success in attaining the four levels of therapy objectives.

Hostility and *suspiciousness* are important barriers to the development of therapeutic trust. Therefore, we examined the relationships among ratings on the BPRS factor hostility, rated at discharge (the period immediately before the initiation of family therapy), drug level, and the level of therapy objectives attained. For this analysis patients were classified as high or low on hostility, based on a median split. The interaction between drug level and hostility at discharge, depicted in Figure 8-2, was highly significant: $F(1, 36) = 9.25$, $p < .005$. This figure indicates that when a patient showed considerable hostility,

Figure 8-2. Mean ratings of highest objective achieved in therapy. The interaction of drug level and BPRS factor *hostility*, rated at time of discharge from inpatient treatment, is illustrated.

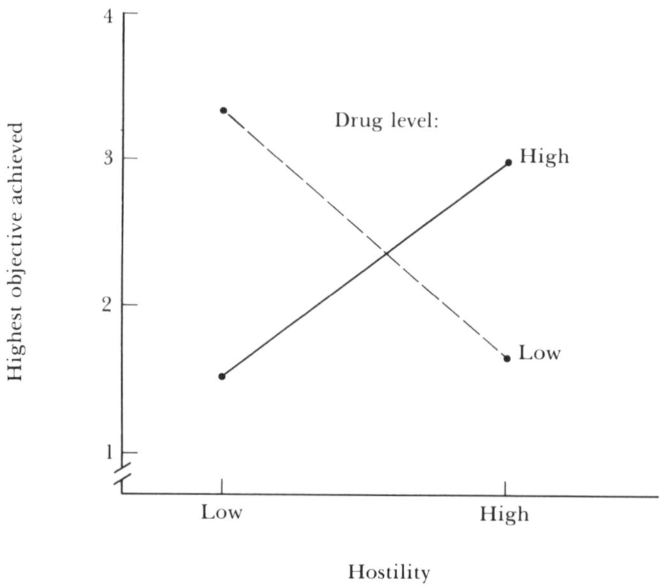

suspiciousness, and uncooperativeness at discharge, therapists indicated that they could achieve the majority of their therapy objectives only when the patient was on the high dose. However, an inverse effect was noted for patients below the median on BPRS hostility at discharge; attainment of therapy objectives was more likely for patients assigned to the low-dose condition. No other BPRS factor score interacted with drug level in predicting the level of therapy objectives attained.

Ratings of Achievement of Objectives as a Predictor Variable. After examining some of the variables which affect ratings of patients' achievement of objectives in therapy, we next determined whether the variance in these ratings related to clinical status at six weeks and at the six-month follow-up period. For these analyses, patients were divided on the basis of a median split on the Guttman scaling of the ratings of achievement of objectives. Patients below the median achieved no higher than objective two and are referred to as nonachievers. Patients above the median achieved objective three or four and are referred to as achievers.

A repeated measure, ANOVA using the Spitzer-Endicott Global Assessment Scale (GAS; Endicott, Spitzer, Fleiss, et al., 1976) ratings at admission, six weeks, and six months, indicates a large improvement for both groups: $F(1, 36)$ for linear trend = 201.5, $p < .005$. However, a significant difference in the slope of the GAS scores was found for achievers and nonachievers of therapy objectives: $F(2,42) = 5.10$, $p < .01$. As Figure 8-3 indicates, patients who were rated as achieving therapy objectives showed greater improvement than did patients who did not achieve objectives. GAS scores were also analyzed separately for each period. There were no significant differences between these groups at admission or at the end of the six weeks, but patients who achieved therapy objectives were rated significantly higher at the six-month follow-up: $F(1,36) = 4.65$, $p < .04$. It appears that the two groups were similar at admission and at the end of treatment. Between the end of the controlled period treatment and the six-month follow-up, patients who were rated as having achieved therapy objectives continued to improve markedly on independent ratings of functioning, while patients who did not achieve higher therapy objectives improved little during this period.

Analyses of the BPRS factor ratings at six weeks and six months were conducted in order to identify the specific symptom clusters which contributed to the greater improvement of patients rated at having achieved therapy objectives. Of the four factors, only *thought disorder*

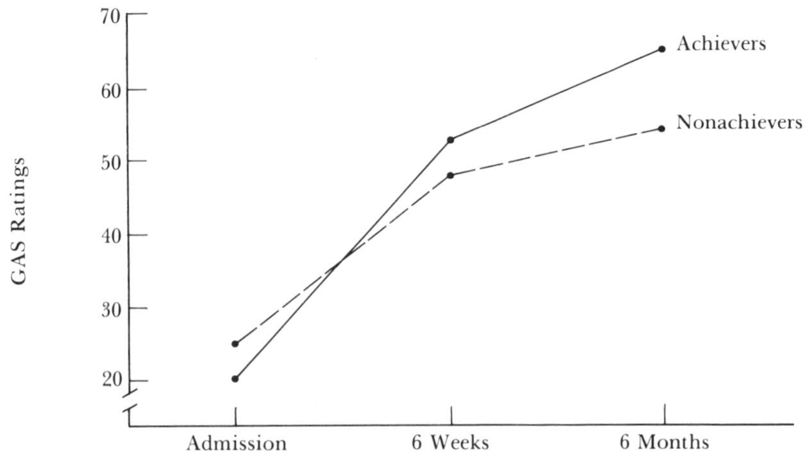

Figure 8-3. Mean Global Assessment Scale (GAS) ratings. Ratings were made at admission, six weeks, and six months for achievers and nonachievers of therapy objectives.

revealed clear differences between achievers and nonachievers. There was no difference between these groups at six weeks, but achievers displayed significantly less thought disorder at six months: $F(1,36) = 8.13$, $p < .01$. Figure 8-4 indicates that patients who were rated as achieving therapy objectives continued to show decreases in thought disorder while patients who did not achieve therapy objectives displayed a tendency for thought disorder to return to prior levels.

Behavioral Correlates of Therapist Ratings of Objectives. The previous analyses indicated that therapists' observations of the degree to which they could deliver the crisis model significantly predicted longer term impact of the therapy, particularly on key symptoms of the schizophrenic process. But, what were therapists reacting to in their ongoing contacts? Evidently, it was something other than classic symptoms of psychopathology. In an effort to get a clearer idea of therapeutic behavior that differentiated achievers from nonachievers, we blindly coded the audio tapes of the therapy sessions.

The coding system drew from many sources, but the most interesting concept came from the work of Vaughn and Leff (1976); they termed it *expressed emotion* (EE), which has been reported to predict relapse in schizophrenics. EE refers to familial attitudes of criticism, hostility, and overinvolvement specifically directed at the identified pa-

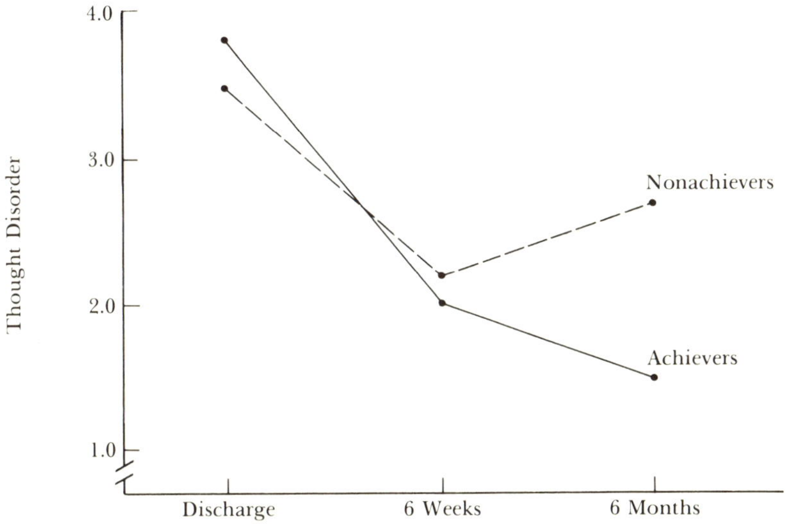

Figure 8–4. Mean *thought disorder* factor scores. The Brief Psychiatric Rating Scale was administered at discharge, six weeks, and six months for achievers and nonachievers of therapy objectives.

tient. Schizophrenics returned to high EE homes have been found to have very high rates of relapse. Codes were developed to mirror the EE components of hostility, criticism, and overinvolvement as they might be expressed in actual family interactions in the therapy tapes. Using tapes from the latter part of the six-session crisis-oriented series, we found that higher levels of EE-type behaviors were observed in nonachiever-rated family units ($p < .002$). Interestingly, the criticism, hostility, and overinvolvement was as likely to be manifested by the patient as by the family member. While this is a gross oversimplification of the data, it does indicate clearly that there are definite behavioral differences observable between families rated as achievers or nonachievers. The differences observed indicate that, late in the course of therapy, high EE-type behaviors were still occurring in the nonachiever group, providing a link between the Vaughn-Leff literature on relapse and the current intervention study. Currently, we are investigating whether these high EE behaviors are present to different degrees in early therapy sessions in achiever and nonachiever samples. If they are, then clearly there are systematic differences between these two types of families which persist throughout six weeks of therapy. If they are not present initially, then it tells us something about possible flaws in the application of the crisis model which are potentially correctable.

Comment

The present study clearly indicates that both phenothiazine medication and a form of family therapy play a significant role in decreasing relapse in acute, young schizophrenics after discharge into the community. In the short run, all therapy receivers showed less residual symptomatology than did patients who did not receive therapy, with the most notable effects being on blunted affect and withdrawal. Over the longer follow-up period, only the therapy receivers who had been maintained at the higher dose level during the six-week control period sustained their earlier gains. We do not know at this time how this delayed effect was achieved—whether high-dose patients were more likely to follow subsequent treatment recommendations or whether this is a genuine delayed effect of a short-term intervention remains to be established.

While all therapy patients showed positive results in terms of emotional withdrawal, impact on other components of the core schizophrenic symptoms were dependent upon the degree of therapist success in delivering the full model of the crisis therapy. These data suggest that there may be two levels of therapy effects, nonspecific and specific. Nonspecific effects are the consequence of maintaining a relationship with the patient and significant others but do not require attainment of all therapy objectives. Such a family support system appears to reduce the affective symptoms associated with the post-acute phase of a schizophrenic episode, such as emotional withdrawal, blunted affect, and, to a lesser degree, anxiety and depression.

Specific therapy effects, on the other hand, require achievement of discrete therapeutic objectives such as those identified by the current crisis model. Achievement of these specific objectives is not necessary for improvement in affective symptoms, but it is critical for sustained improvement in a core symptom of schizophrenia—thought disorder. Signs of the return of thought disorder are evident in patients who did not move beyond step two of the crisis model, while continued attenuation is noted for those who were rated as having attained steps three or four. If we examine the differences between steps one and two and between steps three and four, there is delineated a shift between a past and future time perspective. Patients who are rated as three or four can extrapolate from the immediate, crisis-laden past to develop strategies for dealing with future stresses. When that shift in time orientation is noted, there is sustained improvement for the next six months, not only in the affective symptoms but in thinking as well. These data support the position that, when the schizophrenic individual can integrate the psychotic experience into his life and use this integration in dealing with subsequent life events, a more positive outcome can be anticipated.

References

ASTRACHAN, B.M., HARROW, D., ADLER, D., et al. A checklist for the diagnosis of schizophrenia. *Brit. J. Psychiat., 121:*529–539, 1972.

CHIEN, C., COLE, J.O. Depot phenothiazine treatment in acute psychosis: A sequential comparative clinical study. *Amer. J. Psychiat., 130:*13–18, 1973.

ENDICOTT, J., SPITZER, R.L., FLEISS, J.F., et al. The global assessment procedure for measuring the overall severity of psychiatric disturbance. *Arch. Gen. Psychiat., 33:*766–771, 1976.

EVANS, J.R., GOLDSTEIN, M.J., and RODNICK, E.H. Premorbid adjustment, paranoid diagnosis, and remission in acute schizophrenics treated in a community mental health center. *Arch. Gen. Psychiat., 28:*666–672, 1973.

KING, C., and GOLDSTEIN, M.J. Therapists' ratings of achievement of therapy objectives: An aid to research on psychotherapy with acute schizophrenics. *Schizophrenic Bull., 5:*118–129, 1979.

MAY, P.R.A. The implications of psychopharmacological research for treatment of schizophrenia. In West, L., and Flinn, D. (Eds.), *Treatment of schizophrenia: Progress and prospects.* New York: Grune and Stratton, 1976, pp. 61–77.

———. *Treatment of Schizophrenia.* New York: Science House, 1968.

MOSHER, L.R., POLLIN, W., and STABENAU, J.R. Families with identical twins discordant for schizophrenia: Some relationships between identification, thinking styles, psychopathology, and dominance-submissiveness. *Brit. J. Psychiat., 118:*29–42, 1971.

OVERALL, J.E., and GORHAM, D.R. The brief psychiatric rating scale. *Psychol. Rep., 10:*799, 1962.

SCHOOLER, N.R. Antipsychotic drugs and psychological treatment in schizophrenia. In Lipton, M.A., DiMascio, A., and Killam, K.F. (Eds.), *Psychopharmacology—A generation of progress.* New York: Raven Press, 1978.

VAUGHN, C. E., and LEFF, J.P. The measurement of expressed emotion in families of psychiatric patients. *Brit. J. Soc. Clin. Psychol., 15:*157–165, 1976.

CHAPTER 9

Drug and Psychological Treatment in the Aftercare of Schizophrenia: A Research Odyssey

Gerard E. Hogarty

FACED WITH WHAT APPEARS TO BE a rather academic and most certainly an insurmountable task—the review of drug and social therapy in the treatment of schizophrenia—I've decided to recall for you the odyssey of two human beings: John D. Fictitious and Mary (NMI) Anonymous.

John and Mary are two rather nondescript individuals unknown to any other human beings beyond a small, but equally obscure, network of lay and professional people. Their lives are undistinguished, save for the fact that John and Mary live in a foster home.

Like many others, each day they rise, eat, and engage in a series of perfunctory tasks characterized by uniformity, regimentation, and monotony. Their meals are adequately prepared but taken separately from the foster family. There is little interaction at table. Food is portioned in advance, eliminating the subsequent need to be served or to ask for things to be passed. At the end of meals, each rises to empty his or her own plate. An unzipped fly goes unnoticed by Mary. The residue of gravy left on her mouth and dress seems an insufficient basis for comment by John.

Throughout the week, personal care and grooming, including when to bathe, to shave, or to get one's hair set or cut, are structured by day and by time. Simple chores, such as hanging the wash, are characterized by habituation and the absence of autonomy. Mary carries the clothes to the washer, stands like a sentinel throughout the fifty-minute cycle, waits for the foster mother to empty the wash, and proceeds to the clothes line. John works in "his" garden where the selection of seed, fertilizer, and implements has been made beforehand by the foster father.

Social improprieties go unnoticed by the foster mother, who never criticizes. Pocket money or trips to the community are carefully scheduled and monitored. The "family" goes to church on Sunday morning, where a familiar face sometimes evokes a nod of recognition, but never to the social gathering on Sunday evening.

In the early evening, John and Mary retire to their own sitting room, again separate from that of the foster family. A television set drones its polished message for an hour or two, but otherwise their own silence is only occasionally interrupted by a fragmented response to a familiar face or program. Sitting is interspersed with periods of aimless pacing. When asked, John and Mary refer to each other as "friends," but they seldom talk together, share chores, play games, or even borrow money. They *never* walk together, cry together, laugh together, or sleep together. Lights-out at 9 PM ends a script that most assuredly will be reenacted the following day.

If the story sounds familiar, that is because it reflects in large part the description of foster-care experiences for schizophrenic patients reported by Murphy. On the surface, it is an affront to the humane aftercare philosophy of Fairweather, Sanders, and the Schwartzes, who speak of the need for subcommunities for chronic patients that would encourage social participation and autonomous behavior in an environment that permits failure while learning.

But let's withhold our judgment for a moment; for while it is true that John and Mary are exceptional cases, their uniqueness does *not* lie in the disaster of their personal lives. On the contrary, John's and Mary's foster-care placement represents a *rational* treatment decision that reflects the best empirical evidence drawn from major treatment studies conducted both here and abroad. Unlike the millions who share their illness and whose community treatment reflects the arbitrary "politics of care," including what is available, where human beings are treated, when they are treated, and by whom they are treated, John's and Mary's management is by design. For most, aftercare treatment is influenced as much by fiscal and administrative concerns as by evidence of therapeutic effectiveness. "Treatment," for the most part, is provided by people who have little or no scientific knowledge base regarding the relationship between treatment strategies and patients' needs as these needs are shaped by diagnosis, prognosis, age, sex, race, psychiatric history, family history, and a host of other personal, environmental, and biological determinants. In fact, the social, economic, and interpersonal burdens of schizophrenic disorders are more often borne by the patient's relatives, by public and private welfare agencies, courts, jails, churches, recreation centers, family service agencies, landlords, and bartenders than by foster care programs, day treatment centers, cooperative apartment programs, halfway houses, patient social clubs, social rehabilitation centers, sheltered workshops, transitional work programs, lodges, and the formal individual or group psychotherapies. *But professionals are not to be indicted, for the principles of psychosocial treament of schizophrenia are more like therapeutic roulette than reasoned behavior!* As Phillip May remarked recently following an exquisite review of the treament methods for schizophrenia: "With the exception of drug effect studies, the abundance of opinion and prejudice is equalled only by the dearth of scientific evidence." That conclusion was echoed in the same year by the Group for the Advancement of Psychiatry when they stated: "It is lamentable that major public health decisions about the treament of schizophrenia are being made on the basis of pitifully few studies, and that decisions on educational and treatment programs are not being made on a scientific basis."

So you see, John and Mary are unique because they got to their foster home by choice and not by chance. If you would permit a rather grave injustice to the geography and chronology of major research studies, I'd like to take you through the more important investigations of the past decade or two in which John and Mary had the good fortune to participate, the results of which ultimately determined their rational placement in "Terminal Township," U.S.A.

Years before, while living with each of their families in England, John and Mary had been observed to relapse shortly after hospital discharge. Evidence, which has recently been validated for a third time, suggested that a high level of expressed emotion in their families—that is, an excess of critical comments and/or emotional overinvolvement—was shown to precipitate an exacerbation of symptoms.

Some local critics, negatively disposed toward the influence of environmental factors on the course of schizophrenia, argued that the studies of expressed emotion simply indicate that hostile relatives are more quickly moved to rehospitalize their relatives. These critics ignored the fact that rehospitalization was not the outcome criterion for John and Mary; rather, relapse was the criterion defined as either a change from non-schizophrenic to schizophrenic by Catego criteria (Type I relapse) or a clear and unequivocal exacerbation of symptoms in chronically ill patients (Type II relapse). More than 50 percent of patients living in high EE households relapsed in nine months, a rate which increased to 68 percent if the patient remained in direct face-to-face contact with the offending relative for more than thirty-five hours of each week. Relapse increased to 92 percent in high EE households if the patient were in high contact and not receiving maintenance chemotherapy. Relapse fell dramatically to 15 percent if medication was employed and face-to-face contact were reduced. In "low" expressed emotion households, relapse averaged 13 percent independent of medication or the amount of face-to-face contact.

A reasonable basis for their apparent vulnerability to criticism was established when independent investigators probed the early, subjective, psychotic experiences of John and Mary. It appeared that, at the extremes of arousal, sensory stimuli, particularly of a verbal nature, were capable of evoking profound cognitive and perceptual difficulties, the manifestations of which seemed to involve an inability to filter irrelevant stimuli, to focus attention, and even, at times, a tendency to distort or misinterpret certain words at specific auditory frequencies. These "disperceptions," in turn, were thought to precipitate hallucinations, delusions, loss of ego boundaries, regression, and formal thought disorder as well as such inhibitory and compensatory behavior as withdrawal and blunted affect—the features of schizophrenia. It became clear that many schizophrenic patients, particularly those like John and Mary who had a probable chronic course, could be viewed as being exquisitely sensitive to their environment. As Hirsch commented, they walked a tightrope across the chasm of personal madness from which they could easily be pushed by too little or too much stimulation. Meanwhile, a TransAtlantic Brotherhood of Researchers learned that sensory regulatory functions of the central nervous system, principally those involving the reticular formation and limbic system, seemed deficient in many schizophrenic patients. This observation proved quite compatible with recent evidence of gross brain pathology as well as with related biochemical data which suggested altered neurotransmitter activity or neuroendocrine imbalance, precipitated perhaps by specific enzyme deficiencies, possibly in the critical mesolimbic system. Such irregularity could lead to neuronal excitation capable of producing the regulatory dysfunctions and cognitive and perceptual disturbances that are often described as schizophrenia. As such, John and Mary came to the United States armed with their antipsychotic medication, which was thought to influence multiple receptor sites in the brain, and equipped with the personal knowledge of their specific vulnerability to the environment.

When they landed in California, culture shock precipitated a relapse. In a profound inpatient study of five treatment modalities, the superiority of maintenance chemotherapy in achieving remission and shortening length of hospital stay was again demonstrated over psychotherapy alone, milieu therapy, and electroshock treatment. At approximately the same time, from other centers in the United States, it was learned that most inpatient psychosocial treatments were, in and of themselves, largely ineffective in the absence of chemotherapy. When combined with chemotherapy, selected gains in adjustment were often observed. But inpatient adjustment bore little relationship to length of community stay or to level of community adjustment. There were, of course, some exceptions: long-term hospitalized, drug refractory patients appeared to profit from the "token economy" ward in the absence of chemotherapy. Operant conditioning of delusional and hallucinatory speech and the enhancement of social skills were effective; at times medication could even be titrated against gains made by behavior modification. However, effects seemed highly individual and often failed to generalize to other settings. Further, certain acute schizophrenic patients were observed to do particularly well without medication when treated by experienced psychotherapists, although design errors argued against generalization. Chronic inpatients prepared for community placement were discharged early and were more likely to be employed, which possibly reflected the efforts of staff to discharge research patients early and to find them work—a curious truism.

In the Laingian approach of Soteria House, certain schizophrenic patients were able to resolve their psychoses without medication, but only after four months on the average, in contrast to the unrandomized but medicated controls whose index hospitalization averaged but two weeks. While significantly more controls than experimental subjects relapsed over the next two years (most in the three months following discharge), it would be wise to remember that experimental subjects were still under twenty-four-hour care at Soteria, while their controls were in the community and at risk for relapse. Risk of relapse itself is a function of "time since episode," that is, it decreases with time. The study, however, raises disconcerting questions as to whether a drug-induced remission of psychosis leaves patients more vulnerable to relapse, especially after drug withdrawal, than they might have been had the psychosis been resolved without medication.

Back in the community and on their own, John and Mary suffered periodic exacerbations of symptoms. However, it became clear that many services, including the day hospital, home treatment, residential community placements, and aggressive attempts at community support, could avoid twenty-four-hour inpatient care. But a discouraging trend was also observed; when drugs, supportive social therapy, rehabilitation efforts, or behavioral therapy were withdrawn, performance uniformly decreased. In the case of drug withdrawal, relapse frequently ensued. So John and Mary entered the period of modern psychiatry, one in which they might be able to live the majority of their lives outside the hospital, even though they periodically would become ill.

But how?

Halfway houses were considered, but the frequent criterion of success—avoidance of hospitalization—said little about the quality of adjustment in the community. In fact, among twenty-eight descriptions of halfway houses, only one controlled study of the halfway house as an aftercare resource was available, and this employed a method of questionable validity. Resumption of instrumental role performance was often a significant outcome criterion. On closer inspection, however, descriptions of halfway house samples appear to be testimonials to the good prognostic characteristics of study patients. Further, the goal of most residential facilities is eventual independent living, but it was clear that John and Mary could not live independently, even if they did not require twenty-four-hour inpatient care.

In addition, they were much like the one-third to one-half of chronic patients who were judged to be unable to assume full-time competitive employment. Sheltered workshops seemed indicated, but few that exclusively served the mentally ill were available, in spite of John's and Mary's rather transient existence. Unlike its counterpart in Europe, industry's involvement in the rehabilitation of chronic patients in the United States was thin to say the least, and the occasional "scraps" thrown to rehabilitation efforts were, with few exceptions, mundane, boring, "salvage" operations. While "work" itself was a valid, humane objective, it bore little relationship to clinical status. In fact, it had been shown that working in the open market proved to be an indicator of eventual relapse for many schizophrenic patients, suggesting once again the schizophrenic patients' vulnerability to stress.

Family therapy was another viable treatment approach, but John and Mary, like so many schizophrenic patients, had already been yanked from the bosom of their families by well-intentioned therapists years before. The three existing studies regarding family therapy, however, seemed on the whole to be positive. Langsley's efforts appeared at least to keep certain patients out of the hospital. But most relevant was the study by Goldstein et al. At the end of a controlled six-week treatment phase, and later at six months following discharge (most of the interim period under uncontrolled conditions), no patient receiving family therapy and a standard dosage of fluphenazine enanthate had relapsed, compared to 48 percent of patients in the non-therapy low-dose condition. Other treatment cells averaged 17 percent to 22 percent relapse over six months. A significant main effect for drug therapy and a clear trend for family therapy was observed, but as in other studies that showed no relapse in patients on depot fluphenazine and social therapy, it was difficult to test for an interaction between drug and family therapy—it is tough to do an analysis of variance without any variance. At present, three centers in various parts of the world are demonstrating the ability to forestall relapse among patients who live in high "expressed emotion" households. These approaches share the notion of individual vulnerability to highly stimulating environments. Family therapy is perhaps too strong a term for these interventions; rather, the programs are characterized by a psychoeducational and management approach designed to modify the environmental demands that are often a part of any family's life. In many ways it was unfortunate that John and Mary were not eligible for family therapy. They had become, as it were, live sacrifices on the altar of expediency years before. Families of schizophrenic patients, it seemed, had been viewed etiologically as bad medicine, even though supporting evidence for this belief was indeed thin. The myth persists to this day, since a criterion of success in many studies is separation from family. Too often the chaos in the family of the schizophrenic patient simply reflects their desperate efforts to cope with the behavior of a vulnerable son or daughter for whom the interpersonal and performance necessities of day-to-day existence are unbelievably difficult to negotiate.

John and Mary, ready for life in the community, found themselves in Boston, where they unsuccessfully participated in a controlled study of individual psychotherapy in a specialized milieu. In another unusual hospital experience, they were systematically prepared for cooperative apartment living in the community prior to discharge. While the cooperative apartment program proved useful in maintaining adjustment and avoiding rehospitalization, in order to complete a more ideal existence, John and Mary attended a day treatment center as well. But results were mixed. While hospitalizations of patients followed in the day center were fewer than those maintained in the mental hygiene clinic, John's relatively superior adjustment slipped, while Mary's relatively poor adjustment improved. After six months in the day center, it was hard to distinquish between the progress of the two. At the same time, others who had studied the experience of chronic patients in the day center described "successful" patients as more dependent, less assertive, and more socially incompetent following treatment. The day treatment center was terminated for John and Mary, and they looked wistfully at the recent results from a multi-center collaborative study by Linn et al.

This study indicated that, while relapse in the day treament center was no different over two years from relapse among patients randomly assigned to a medication clinic, the social adjustment of day treatment center patients was significantly improved. However, marked interactions between day center and outcome were observed. Patients treated in the more dynamic day treatment centers (that is, those which had more individual psychotherapy hours, more group therapy, and more private interviewing rooms) were doing poorly; and those patients treated in less dynamic but more structured occupational/recreational programs were doing better. With no clear treatment options available to John and Mary, now or in the past, the risk in entering a dynamic center would have been too much to bear; besides, neither of them was a veteran.

Finally, they moved to Baltimore, after having learned from a New England colleague that Hogarty and his collaborative group were about to begin an aftercare study in which both drug and social therapy experiences would be controlled for the first time. Fortunately, neither

John nor Mary was randomly assigned to placebo alone or to social therapy alone—for *80 percent* of those patients relapsed during the two years of treatment! Among the few lucky survivors on social therapy or placebo alone, those receiving only social therapy (social casework and vocational rehabilitation) were more impaired in their social and personal adjustments than those few patients who were able to survive on placebo alone. Unfortunately, it took eighteen months for the combined effect of drug and social therapy to manifest itself.

In short, these results once again evoked images of the TransAtlantic Brotherhood and their message of stimulus sensitivity. John received drug therapy alone, which further demonstrated his need for medication; he was one of the 52 percent of patients able to survive for a two-year period of time, but his adjustment was unaffected. That is, it was impossible to detect a difference in adjustment between drug and placebo receivers among nonrelapsed patients. Mary received both drug and social therapy and not only avoided relapse, but her personal and social adjustment was significantly improved over the results from drug therapy alone.

Further, it was clear that certain withdrawn, disorganized, anxious, and low-insight patients relapsed more quickly when assigned to social therapy than when assigned to a control condition, validating a prediction based on the *pretreatment characteristics* of patients and not contaminated by patients who survive for selected periods of time, as is erroneously claimed by certain reviewers.

To support the argument that the high relapse rate of patients on drug therapy and a delayed effect of social therapy might be due to drug noncompliance, another study was begun comparing oral and parenteral fluphenazine with or without social therapy. In a provocative finding, recently replicated both here and in England, relapse rates of patients on oral and depot medication remained high and were nearly identical in the first year following hospital discharge; 35 to 40 percent of patients had relapsed by the end of one year. Over the two years of study, there was no difference in relapse rate between oral and depot forms of medication. When noncompliance was circumvented by depot fluphenazine and social therapy was employed, an interactive effect of the combined treatment in forestalling relapse was observed, at least at the .07 level. This result reflected the fact that no patient relapsed between eight and twenty-four months following discharge, a finding reminiscent of Goldstein's family therapy and depot fluphenazine condition.

Eventually the money ran out and these studies ended. John and Mary were again lost in a nonsystem of aftercare and found their way back to the hospital. Here a careful appraisal of their past histories and treatment responses led to their current foster home placement.

When Murphy came to the foster home, he felt that John's and Mary's social adjustments were inferior to the twenty-eight matched controls back at the hospital, but his finding might have reflected more a relatively enriched hospital program or the profound problems associated with matched control groups. Directly following him were Linn et al., who, for the first time in hundreds of years of foster care, randomly assigned patients to foster care or to continued hospitalization. While it was originally believed that John and Mary would be happier in their foster home, they were no more personally comfortable than were their colleagues back at the hospital. But surprisingly, John and Mary and their fellow patients at the four other centers showed considerable improvement in their social adjustment in comparison with hospital controls, even though their levels of performance would not set the world afire. By design, John and Mary found their current foster home. Had they been assigned to a more active foster home, their chances of relapsing again would have increased.

So here they spend their lives as successfully maintained community residents of Terminal Township. If their luck had only held a while longer, it might have brought them to one of twelve or so cities in the United States that has an operating social rehabilitation center—a model of the ideal subcommunity which provides a combination of residential, social, and vocational experiences in the context of autonomous, social participation. Unfortunately, only one controlled study of the social rehabilitation center could be found that clearly indicated success for patients—if they managed to participate in the program. It seemed likely that John and Mary, with the hard-won knowledge of their own vulnerability to the environment, would not have returned to the social rehabilitation center after a single visit. Like most community treatment programs, the limited availability of service is only part of the problem; the major difficulty is one of getting schizophrenic patients to utilize what meager resources do exist, since noncompliance and insight deficiency seem as much a characteristic of the illness as is formal thought disorder.

In their peripatetic existence it was, in many ways, unfortunate that they had not become ill in India, Colombia, or Nigeria. Course and outcome—at least among patients meeting Catego criteria for schizophrenia in the WHO-IPSS study—were better in *developing* countries than in such developed areas as London, Moscow, or Washington, D.C. John reminded me, however, that there was not much call for shepherds in Terminal Township.

When I last visited John and Mary, we spoke of the fact that their medication clinic was soon to begin a relaxed, informal get-together once a month for people like themselves. In the past decade or two, I pointed out, no fewer than nine studies of group and individual aftercare treatment had been conducted. Although scant evidence existed to affirm its value, echoing inpatient studies, the slowly paced, nondynamic, reality-based, informal group offered distinct advantages over individual therapy for role modeling, mutual support, and a level of social stimulation that provided self-regulated participation. I was sure that John's and Mary's characteristic indifference to my proposal could be worked through by the clinic staff who had carefully nurtured a relationship of trust and mutual regard with them over the past few years, a relationship that could be used in times of crises and life change. But they would have to wait for assurance of efficacy, since conclusive evidence on group versus individual differences was yet to be accepted.

Both John and Mary had their own reservations about my proposal which had arisen from their years of participating in formal research programs. They pressed me to summarize, if I could, what the results of their long experience had meant to me, personally, and to the scientific community in general. I rather froze at the seemingly innocuous challenge. The response, however, did come slowly; it was a formulation which, in my heart, I felt best summarized the state of the art regarding drug and social therapy in the aftercare treatment of schizophrenic patients. The statement, however, was more difficult to present than I had imagined. Somewhere there seemed a reasoned path between the "search after meaning," which so often characterizes the reviews of optimists in the field, and the syndrome of pessimism, which either cites the negative findings of uncontrolled studies or views marginal tests of significance and errors in the design of combined studies as the fodder of unjustified despair.

Finally, I began. At one level it seemed that the external environment, however broadly or narrowly defined, did impinge on the course and outcome of certain schizophrenic patients, sometimes positively, sometimes negatively. Negative effects, it should be remembered, are not without their value; they imply that nondrug treatments do exert a powerful influence. It is our ignorance of discrete patient subtypes and their underlying pathogenesis that conspires against a rational joining of available treatments and patient needs. Difficulty in assessing main and interactive effects of nondrug treatments on the course of schizophrenia seemed, in large measure, to be traced to the overwhelming heterogeneity among the group of behaviors that we label schizophrenic. Even when psychosocial effects have been observed, some critics have argued that they do not touch the core of the disorder—an unfair indictment of aftercare treatment. By definition, aftercare seeks to maintain and sustain a remission of core symptoms and to improve the residual performance deficits that so often characterize our patients. Even drug treatment that sustains a remission of symptoms for many patients does little or nothing to resolve deficit symptoms or promote social restoration. Social therapies by themselves, as well, seem to have no specific effect in sustaining patients but, depending on the type of patient, might shorten or lengthen survival time for discrete types. Combined treatment does seem to have some effect, even if not an overwhelming one, in forestalling a relapse and enhancing adjustment; again, this applies to certain poorly defined patients. There is no evidence that chemotherapy interferes with, or otherwise impedes, the effects of psychosocial forms of intervention. Regarding placebo receivers, it is clear that 30 to 35 percent of these patients relapse who would otherwise have been maintained on medication! Unfortunately, an equal number of patients (a number which increases to nearly 50 percent by the two-year mark) relapse *in spite* of guaranteed medication, even though the same drug facilitated the resolution of an earlier acute psychosis. Evidence is now accumulating in support of the fact that personal vulnerability and environmental demands represent the two-edged sword that consigns such patients to periodic psychosis.

At a broad program level, cumulative evidence from uncontrolled and naturalistic studies does seem to indicate a psychostatic quality of social programs, much like the psychostatic quality of drugs described by Heinz Lehman years ago. This means that psychosocial programs are often effective in preventing deterioration and maintaining adjustment.

In many programs, it appears that a significant minority of patients get worse. John interrupted and identified what might well be the dilemma of the 1980s. He noted that, when his performance was good, his symptoms and chance for relapse seemed to increase. When his primary symptoms were in remission and demands were low, his social functioning decreased and remained low as well; this called to mind the work of

Wing, Lamb, and others that implicated understimulating environments in the pathogenesis of negative symptoms. Mary wondered whether the attempts to enhance her social adjustment were fair, if the price, so to speak, was periodic madness. She asked if this wasn't a question that lawyers or theologians and other Great Thinkers should be discussing, rather than mere medical folk.

John added that he often wondered how long he would need medication, since it seemed to him that over time, increasing dosages of medication were being used—reflecting a profound clinical concern about the possibility of increased receptor development or sensitivity over time. I suggested that some slight evidence was available which indicated that dosage requirements might be less in supportive psychosocial programs or within benign environments, but that low dose should not be equated with no dose. In fact, a review of all controlled drug trials in the aftercare of schizophrenic patients indicated a relapse rate on placebo of 68 percent whether the drug was withdrawn at two months or two years following hospital discharge. While 35 to 40 percent of patients relapsed while on drug therapy in the first year post discharge, the rate of relapse is reduced to 12 to 15 percent in subsequent years or among stabilized patients. The neurological risk/prophylactic benefit ratio indeed seemed the contemporary treatment dilemma during the latter part of the twentieth century. Tragically, only one aftercare dosage study has been reported, that of Goldstein, although three other projects are currently in progress.

At this point, John and Mary had that glaze of bewilderment in their eyes; they were obviously reluctant to press their yet fully answered question. I surmised that their unwillingness to interrupt was likely in response to my apparent difficulty in synthesizing the results of their considerable experience. Yielding to a quiet desperation, John finally asked, "But has our participation helped you at all in understanding what's wrong with us now and whether the quality of our lives could be changed for the better in years to come?"

It seemed to me, I surmised, that twenty years of research has begun to suggest certain models for the likely pathogenesis of diverse schizophrenic disorders. One model involved the concepts of arousal, disattention, distraction, and disease, perhaps as the manifestation of some impaired but underlying neurophysiologic, biochemical, or neuroendocrinologic substrate. This model, at least, appears to accommodate both the schizophrenic patient's sensitivity to the stimulation from their inner and outer worlds and the action of antipsychotic drugs, an action that appears to regulate arousal levels and redeploy attention. In this regard, then, maintenance chemotherapy currently lowers but does not eliminate the sensitive patient's vulnerability to the complex, vague, and often excessive developmental and emotional demands of both the therapeutic and natural environments. Effective forms of psychosocial treatment, in turn, become increasingly like personalized exercises in human engineering, enabling patients to structure, modify, and otherwise cope with environmental requirements, while the underlying processes remain under the variable control of medication.

After a moment of uneasy silence, I volunteered to John and Mary that much of their concern about the past application of drug and social therapy reflected a practice that resembled alchemy. I hoped that my summary gave reason to be hopeful, for some recent evidence concerning the characteristics of patients and their environments did give promise of treatment specificity. It was becoming clear, from work underway, that one could stay on the tightrope of sanity and improve adjustment as well if the opportunity to learn slowly in a structured, stimulus-modulated environment was made available. What was needed, however, were more specific indicators of diagnostic specificity, personal vulnerability, and environmental vulnerability. Some hope existed that such traditional measures of personal vulnerability as attention and arousal deficits, test dose responses, EEG parameters, and family history, for example, might serve as indicators of treatment response, course, and outcome. Refined measures of the therapeutic and natural environments of patients could, in turn, be tested for interactions in this psychosocial-biological model. The model at least held promise of ultimately binding available treatments to individual patient needs.

Mary asked whether this was ever to be a reality—or would remain a shared fantasy of patients and professionals. "A fantasy, unfortunately," I answered, "unless the following objectives could be achieved: (1) a more consistent policy of funding research regarding psychosocial factors and the combined treatment of schizophrenic conditions beyond the rate of $125,000 in new money available in 1975 at the federal level or the $1 million in 1978 and without the threatened reduction of funds in 1980—funding practices at the federal level over the past ten years have promoted a form of "scientificus interruptus," a system which undermines the rights of researchers, clinicians, and patients themselves, both now and in the future; (2) more complete education of clinicians and researchers alike—at the moment, standard treatment texts available to *allied* professionals, for example, too often ignore data on pathogenesis, decry diagnosis, and present selected and frequently biased reviews of the treatment literature; (3) closely related is the need for more adequate training programs for people interested in careers in clinical research—at the moment, clinical research suffers a variation of Catch 22; investigators are infrequently supported because their applications are weak, and applications are weak because investigators lack training, but there is little money for training because applications for training funds are themselves weakly developed; (4) more research with appropriate controls is needed and less so-called program evaluation, a strategy often used synonymously with research but in essence representing a conspiracy to make the world safe for politicians and administrators; as such, there must be far more hypothesis testing and less hypothesis generating; finally, (5) much more attention must be paid by clinicians and researchers alike to current diagnostic and current etiologic theories with their attending implications for treatment. A clear move away from the problem-oriented individual case approach is a necessity."

By this time, Mary began to stare off into space and quietly placed her hands over her ears. John remarked that all this was a bit too much for him and that it seemed now that two or three people were speaking the same message at the same time.

No, I thought, it's more than two or three voices, but not the thousands needed to formulate a stable policy regarding funding of training programs, services, and research, although it did seem believable that a few thousand people could clearly influence the few hundred elected representatives at local and federal levels.

I concluded with a good night to John, a good night to Mary, and a reminder that the lights were going out soon.

Echoing my farewell, they added, "And good luck with your New York Conference crowd."

"And to you, John and Mary," I replied, "because luck is what you will truly need if the light of wisdom that comes with systematic inquiry really does go out!"

References

The relevant literature so lightly cited can be identified in the following sources:

ANDERSON, C.M., HOGARTY, G.E., and REISS, D.J. Family treatment of adult schizophrenic patients: A research based psycho-educational approach. *Schizophrenia Bull.*, *6*; 3 (1980), 490–505.

Schizophrenia Bull., *6;* 1 (1980) (entire issue).

CHAPTER 10

Psychotherapeutic Attitudes in the Drug Treatment of Anxiety and Phobic Reactions

Donald F. Klein and
Michael R. Liebowitz

Our discussion will focus on phobic anxiety, listed in the Diagnostic and Statistical Manual (DSM-III) as Panic Disorder with Agoraphobia. As background we will present an illustrative case, followed by a discussion of the phenomenology and drug treatment of this disorder. We will then go on to review research findings and conceptual issues regarding supportive, behavioral, and psychoanalytic psychotherapy approaches to phobic anxiety in the context of drug treatment. While focusing principally on one clinical condition, we hope to provide a conceptual and methodological framework applicable to evaluating psychotherapeutic approaches joined with drug treatment in a variety of psychiatric syndromes.

This research was supported in part by NIMH grants MH-30906 and MH-33422.

Presentation of Case

Introduction and Chief Complaint

The patient is a thirty-two-year-old, married female magazine editor, referred to the Depression Evaluation Service of the New York State Psychiatric Institute and Columbia Presbyterian Medical Center by her internist for psychiatric evaluation and treatment of recurrent severe anxiety attacks.

Present Illness

The patient reported that for the past six months she had experienced frequent episodes of severe anxiety. These episodes would start without identifiable precipitants, build up "like a wave" to a level of panic over fifteen to twenty minutes, and gradually subside by the end of an hour. When having these attacks, the patient reported the following: "My chest tightens, my ears clog, my palms sweat, I have a sense of dread, and it feels like I'm losing control." These episodes occurred in a variety of situations, especially where rapid exit was difficult, such as supermarket lines, buses, crowded stores, restaurants, and elevators. In each case the patient would immediately cease what she was doing and flee the situation, even if it meant, for example, abandoning a basket full of groceries she was waiting to pay for. Furthermore, she had begun to limit her activities because she feared having a panic attack. Thus, she avoided restaurants and department stores, took taxis instead of buses, and shopped at times when there were no lines in the supermarkets.

She had seen her internist several times for this problem. He had prescribed diazepam (Valium) 10 mg TID for her anxiety symptoms, which calmed her between episodes but did not block the panic attacks. She was on no other medication. She denied use of other psychoactive agents or abuse of alcohol.

The patient had been upset and worried by her elderly father's declining health over the past year. She had also suffered a spontaneous abortion eight months before her anxiety symptoms began, after developing preeclampsia in her sixth month of pregnancy. Finally, she had experienced several weeks of unrelenting criticism by her superior at work in the period immediately prior to the onset of her panic attacks.

Her first panic attack occurred during a business luncheon, from which she had to hastily excuse herself. Because of her boss's constant criticism and refusal to grant her vacation time to visit her ailing father, she quit her job, stayed at home without working for three months, and then took a less-demanding job, all without resolution of her symptoms.

She also began to feel depressed after several months, with a loss of enthusiasm for life, accompanied by initial insomnia and a fifteen-pound weight loss; this lasted for approximately two months. She had regained the weight by the time of her initial psychiatric consultation, although her initial insomnia persisted. In addition, her abilities to enjoy friends, sex, reading, television, and other activities were at no time impaired. She denied middle or terminal insomnia, loss of energy, symptoms of agitation or psychomotor retardation, self-reproach or inappropriate guilt feelings, diurnal variation, inability to concentrate or make decisions, or recurrent thoughts about death or suicide.

Past Psychiatric History

The patient had experienced one prior panic attack several years earlier when trapped in a malfunctioning elevator. She had no prior history of psychiatric disorder and had never previously consulted a psychiatrist. She had, however, for most of her adult life felt somewhat uncomfortable in crowds and in certain situations from which ready exit was difficult. As an example, she noted that she would habitually sit on the outside of a luncheonette booth rather than on the inside. She had almost been despondent for several weeks after her spontaneous abortion, but this response was without vegetative signs and with prompt return to normal function.

Social History

The patient is the oldest of five siblings, the other four of whom were male, born to an established small-town family. The only family history of diagnosed psychiatric disorder was a long stay in a sanitarium by her paternal grandmother for a nervous breakdown and a tendency for her father to abuse alcohol occasionally.

The patient described her childhood as happy. She had no difficulty leaving home for school or summer camp. The family was economically secure and socially well placed. Her parents got along reasonably well.

The patient's father was overseas in military service at the time of her birth and did not return home until after her second birthday. He is reported to have been verbally abusive to his children at times when he had had too much to drink, criticizing their intelligence and challenging them to argue back and defend themselves. The patient would fight back more than would her siblings, but she felt at such times that she was in a no-win situation, since her father liked to argue and to outwit his children and would never admit he was wrong. Thus the arguments would continue until the children submitted—the only way to regain their father's affection. In general, the patient felt that she and her siblings had to humor their father to maintain his affection and approval. If they didn't humor him, they had to stay out of his way.

There appeared to be no unusual problems in adolescence, either academic or social. She attended a highly rated college, went on to obtain a graduate degree, married a successful businessman, and settled in a large city. She worked for several years in public relations, finally quitting because she felt that male co-workers were being advanced more quickly than she. She then became an editor of a magazine, during which time she became pregnant for the first time, developed toxemia, and miscarried. She went back to the same job, but after several months she started to feel unfairly, unrelentingly criticized by her boss. At this point her panic symptoms began.

Medical History

The patient had a post-traumatic splenectomy during her mid-twenties. The only other pertinent medical history is described in the present illness.

The patient had had a full, normal work-up by her internist, including physical examination and laboratory evaluation, immediately prior to her referral.

Mental Status

The patient was a slender, fashionably dressed woman who looked her stated age and appeared worried about her symptoms, distressed by their restrictive effect on her life, and bewildered as to why they were happening. She was sad without psychomotor retardation. There was no psychotic ideation or cognitive impairment. She related in a cooperative and appropriate manner.

Diagnosis

In terms of DSM-II, this patient would have been diagnosed as having features of an anxiety neurosis, a phobic neurosis, and a depressive neurosis. In DSM-II an anxiety neurosis was characterized by anxious overconcern—extending to panic and frequently associated with somatic symptoms such as faintness or palpitations—that would occur under any circumstances. A patient with a phobic neurosis might show similar symptoms, but only when exposed to specific situations or objects that were consciously recognized as presenting no real danger. Phobias were generally attributed to fears displaced to the phobic situation or object from some other source of which the person was unaware.

Clinical research findings of the past two decades, however, now permit us more precisely to dissect these anxiety and phobic conditions. For example, the patient discussed above began to have brief episodes of intense anxiety or panic six months before presenting for psychiatric treatment. These episodes characteristically began spontaneously or "out of the blue," building in intensity until they were intolerable. While first occurring at a business luncheon, the panic attacks soon began to happen on supermarket lines, buses, crowded stores, restaurants, and elevators. Whenever they occurred, she was forced to flee the situation precipitously before her anxiety symptoms would abate. It is interesting to note that this patient, like others, had mild claustrophobic symptoms for years before the onset of her panic attacks.

Within a short time the patient began to feel anxious before entering the above-mentioned situations—that is, she began to worry that she might become panicky. She was thus experiencing anticipatory anxiety when she had to be in a supermarket, restaurant, bus, or elevator. The third and final step was to begin

> to avoid the feared situations, to develop phobic avoidance of places in which panic attacks had occurred; this seemed to include any situation in which immediate exit was difficult or access to trusted persons restricted.

The crucial distinction to be made is that the core event was the spontaneous panic attacks, which led to the development of anticipatory anxiety and then phobic avoidance. That the panic attack is qualitatively distinct from, and not just an intensification of, the anticipatory anxiety is supported by their differential pharmacological responsivity. Klein (1964) demonstrated that the panic attacks *themselves* could be blocked by the tricyclic antidepressant imipramine, which, however, did not immediately affect the anticipatory anxiety and the subsequent avoidant behavior. Benzodiazepines and other minor tranquilizers, on the other hand, ameliorated the anticipatory anxiety but had no effect on the panic attacks themselves. Thus, panic attacks appear to represent a form of anxiety biologically distinct from anticipatory (or free-floating) anxiety.

This in turn leads to a more logical classification of phobic disorders, with a separation of those involving spontaneous panic attacks from those that do not. Agoraphobia, or a fear of open or public places, is most often actually a fear of leaving home, based in turn on a fear of having a panic attack. The panic attacks themselves are often episodic and may abate spontaneously after six to twelve months. However, they tend to be recurrent and occasionally become chronic. In addition, the agoraphobic behavior often becomes chronic because the patient may eventually give up trying to enter feared situations.

Other types of phobias that do not involve spontaneous panic attacks may include simple conditioned phobias (post-traumatic avoidances) such as the avoidance of large dogs after being bitten by one, the avoidance of feared objects that may have a symbolic or unconscious meaning, and social phobias, which involve fears of eating or speaking in public, meeting new people, and so forth, and which may involve issues of low self-esteem as well as previous conditioning. As will become clear, the presence or absence of spontaneous panic attacks has crucial treatment implications.

The first episode of panic attacks occurs in many patients, especially females, upon either threatened or actual separation from or loss of a loved person. Such patients often have histories of childhood separation anxiety as well. In one such study, 20 percent of outpatients and 50 percent of inpatients with panic disorder had histories of childhood separation anxiety, which was often manifested as difficulty in attending school (Klein, 1964).

A common precipitant for male patients is a life-threatening event or illness. Another substantial proportion of patients seems to develop panic attacks in the context of endocrinological change. In a grouping of thirty-two patients, panic attacks began in three patients within a year of oophorectomy; in three within a year of hysterectomy; in three within one month postpartum; in two within a week prepartum; and in one within a week after beginning thyroid supplements as treatment for hypothyroidism with associated amenorrhea (Klein, 1964). The patient reported in our case study had a miscarriage and toxemia eight months before the onset of her panic attacks. Thus some phobic-anxious patients appear to have a lifelong vulnerability to separation-induced anxiety, while others have normal life adjustments until the onset of their anxiety symptoms following a traumatic life event or alteration of endocrine status (Klein, 1964).

Despite the diversity of precipitating events, all patients with spontaneous panic attacks may have a common pathophysiological aberration. As was first pointed out by Pitts and McClure (1967) and later replicated by Fink, Taylor, and Volavka (1970), it is possible to precipitate panic attacks routinely, in patients prone to spontaneous episodes of panic, by the intravenous administration of sodium lactate. This does not occur in more than 10 percent of normals, who for the most part experience rather mild symptomatology such as slight paresthesias and muscle tremor. Furthermore, spontaneous panic attacks can be blocked by two distinct types of antidepressant drugs—the tricyclics imipramine and desmethylimipramine, and the monoamine oxidase inhibitor phenelzine (Klein, 1964; Klein and Fink, 1962).

The recognition that certain drugs specifically block panic attacks was a major breakthrough in the treatment of anxiety and phobic disorders. Until that time, the treatment of agoraphobic patients with panic attacks was usually based on the premise that such individuals required extended outpatient psychotherapies devoted to an exploration of unconscious sexual and aggressive impulses, the phobically barred areas being interpreted as symbolizing forbidden temptations. However, while patients given imipramine or phenelzine reported a dramatic decrease or cessation of panic attacks, many were still reluctant to change their phobic-avoidant behavior patterns. Persuasion, direction, support, and/or minor tranquilizers were often required *after the panic at-*

tacks had been blocked to help patients alleviate their anticipatory anxiety, which was not ameliorated directly by the antipanic effects of the drugs, and thus allow them to return to the phobically avoided situations.

Once it has been ascertained that a patient is suffering spontaneous panic attacks and other medical and psychiatric conditions are excluded, a trial of imipramine is warranted. However, the role of support and of urging patients to reenter avoided situations after the panic attacks are pharmacologically blocked cannot be overstressed. In this regard the therapist must educate patients as to the distinctions between panic attacks, anticipatory anxiety, and phobic avoidance. The therapist must also help overcome demoralization by explaining that most people would act the same way in the face of panic attacks and that the patient's reaction pattern is not a sign of weakness or cowardliness. One must stress that the panic attacks can be pharmacologically blocked and that, however high their anticipatory anxiety, patients will then be able to enter feared situations without experiencing panic. Anything that facilitates this process is helpful, and if other measures fail, minor tranquilizers can be used to moderate anticipatory anxiety. Finally, one must be readily available, on a twenty-four hour basis, to calm fears raised by medication side effects as well as by occasional panic attacks that break through in an inadequately medicated patient.

The role of specific behavior therapy techniques alone, or in conjunction with pharmacotherapy, is less clear. Zitrin et al. (1978) conducted a twenty-six-week study of behavior therapy plus imipramine, behavior therapy plus placebo, and supportive psychotherapy plus imipramine in patients classified as agoraphobics, simple phobics, or mixed phobics. The supportive psychotherapy was dynamically oriented and nondirective, while the behavior therapy consisted of relaxation training, systematic desensitization in imagination, specific in vivo desensitization homework assignments, and assertiveness training in addition to supportive therapy. The agoraphobics all suffered panic attacks, while the simple phobics had discrete phobias such as claustrophobia, fear of animals, social phobias, and so on. The mixed phobics had spontaneous panic attacks but only circumscribed phobias with no travel restrictions. The great majority of patients in all groups showed moderate to marked global improvement (70 to 86 percent, depending on the rater). In agoraphobics and mixed phobics (both groups experiencing spontaneous panic attacks), imipramine was significantly superior to placebo. There was no difference between the effects of behavior therapy and supportive psychotherapy, both resulting in high improvement rates (76 percent to 100 percent, depending on the rater). Simple phobics showed a high rate of improvement with all treatment regimens (72 to 93 percent, depending on the rater), with no significant difference between imipramine and placebo or between behavior therapy and supportive therapy.

The lack of superiority of behavior therapy over supportive therapy is striking in this study, particularly for the simple phobia group for whom there was no imipramine benefit to complicate the comparison of psychotherapies. One explanation may be that patients who came to the Phobia Clinic, where the study was being conducted, were highly motivated to improve and would often themselves initiate attempts to enter a phobic situation while attributing the initiative to their therapists. Thus a patient might say: "Perhaps it's about time I tried riding a bus." The therapist using a nondirective, supportive approach would say: "It sounds like you think it's time to try a bus ride." The patient might then respond: "You think it's time I tried a bus ride. Yes, I'll do as you say and try it."

"Trying it" seems the key to successful treatment, and anything that facilitates that seems helpful. One technique that has been used to accomplish this is a group exposure in vivo, first applied to agoraphobics by Hand et al. (1974). In another study by Klein's group at Hillside, seventy-six agoraphobic women were treated with combined group exposure in vivo and imipramine or placebo in a randomized double-blind study (Zitrin, Klein, and Woerner, 1980). Groups of patients accompanied by a therapist would enter phobic situations; therapy consisted of ten weekly sessions lasting three to four hours each. The format consisted of a therapist meeting with the group for forty-five minutes of discussion and then accompanying them into phobic situations. The therapist served as a group leader who was supportive yet authoritative and took a firm, insistent stance in regard to group members entering and remaining in phobic situations until their anxiety subsided. Patients' initial tasks consisted of walking alone from the hospital to a shopping center six city blocks away, entering and remaining in a large department store, with each patient in a different department of the store, and eating lunch in a restaurant. Then, each patient walked back to the hospital alone.

In subsequent sessions, patients were required to drive to more distant shopping centers; enter crowded stores; travel alone by bus, train, and subway; and, in the final stage of treatment, travel alone into the heart of New York City (Manhattan). There they repeated the experience of entering crowded stores, entered other crowded areas of the city, had lunch in a crowded restaurant, and then traveled back to the hospital area alone on the subway. To reinforce the effects of the treatment sessions, patients were requested to repeat the session experiences as homework assignments.

In our view, in vivo exposure, as done in our clinic, is more akin to in vivo desensitization than to in vivo flooding, because we do not immediately put patients into situations that are at the top of the fear hierarchy. If this were truly a flooding procedure, it would be necessary in the very first session to insist that they take the subway alone to Manhattan and spend at least an hour in a crowded department store. Instead, we defer that kind of exposure until the latter part of treatment. Furthermore, we do not deliberately try to induce anxiety. At all times, the patient controls the amount of anxiety to which he or she is willing to be exposed, albeit under therapist and group pressure.

A majority of the patients in both the imipramine and the placebo groups showed moderate to marked improvement. However, imipramine was significantly superior to placebo on three of the four reported measures of improvement—primary phobia, spontaneous panic, and global improvement. A comparison of these patients with those previously treated with imipramine and imaginal desensitization showed a superiority of exposure in vivo midway in treatment, that is, after fourteen weeks, but no significant difference between groups at the completion of therapy (after twenty-six weeks). This disadvantage of exposure in vivo is that there are certain patients who simply will not or cannot tolerate the technique; hence we encountered a 29 percent dropout rate for this approach as opposed to an 18 percent dropout rate for imaginal desensitization. It would appear that patients who can respond to exposure in vivo are a highly self-selected group who are more highly motivated and less frightened than those who accept less arduous therapies.

Another group of investigators (Matthew, Johnston, Lancashire, et al., 1976) using behavioral techniques have reported that there are no long-term differences between the effects of treatments involving exposure to imagined or real situations as long as patients are encouraged to practice between sessions. They also note that all of their patients identified as the main therapeutic effect the therapists' encouragement and sympathy. It is our experience as well that the patient-therapist relationship, including transference factors and the therapeutic alliance, appears to be a powerful force in persuading patients to confront phobic situations, with or without explicit instructions by therapists to do so. These features are particularly heightened in specialized phobia clinics, which patients often perceive as their last resort and therefore endow with a certain "Lourdes-like" quality, which may account for the high success rates such facilities have, even in patients failing to benefit from treatment in less charismatic settings. This willingness to enter phobic situations is an essential ingredient in the successful treatment of phobias, especially if panic attacks can be prevented, while doing so, by concomitant drug therapy.

What, then, of helping the patient to understand the evolution of his phobic anxiety in terms of his particular interpersonal and intrapsychic functioning? In the case presented in this report, it appears that the patient began to experience panic attacks when subjected to intense criticism by her boss, a situation that may have reactivated childhood conflicts in dealing with an autocratic father. With the panic attacks pharmacologically suppressed and the patient once again able to function at her normal level, we initiated a psychotherapeutic exploration of this issue. Ultimately the patient's ability to be more appropriately assertive with male authority figures was enhanced. One might thus hypothesize a psychodynamic component in the onset of her panic attacks. One could also speculate, however, that the change in endocrine status following her miscarriage created the patient's vulnerability to the panic attacks, or set the stage, as it were, requiring only a nonspecific environmental stress to initiate the clinical syndrome. In general, the specific role of psychological issues in both the etiology and treatment of panic attacks and agoraphobia are quite unclear. It is this area that we would now like to discuss.

The traditional psychodynamic understanding is that agoraphobic individuals have failed in their attempts to cope with conflicted sexual or aggressive impulses by repression. Instead, they displace their conflict onto places or situations in the outside world that stimulate these impulses; if the mechanism works, their anxiety is then encapsulated and confined to those situations. If such places can be avoided, anxiety is ameliorated, and this avoidance is seen as the essence of agoraphobia (MacKinnon and Michels, 1971).

An example used to support this formulation is the case of a woman afraid to walk in the street by herself. In her initial interviews with a psychiatrist, she denied awareness of what she feared, saying only that she might become upset if she tried to walk in the street alone. Somewhat later she verbalized that some man might make sexual advances toward her. Only much later in treatment she reported the recognition that she feared that she might not decline such overtures. Thus the refusal to walk in the street alone is seen as a way of avoiding sexual temptation without recognition by the patient of the actual sexual conflict. Concurrently, infantile and dependent wishes are gratified by the insistence on always being accompanied outside the home.

An alternative explanation of this sequence, however, is that the patient, desperate to find a reason for having what was really an unprecipitated panic attack, was willing to accept and elaborate the explanation of unconscious sexual conflict after it was suggested by her therapist.

This vignette was initially offered as an example of displacement without symbolization—that is, the patient shifted her attention from an emotional conflict to the environment in which the conflict occurred. More elaborate displacements are said to be based on symbolic representation, such as a fear of driving a car into a tunnel or riding on a subway because they symbolically represent the act of sexual intercourse.

Finally, displacements are also thought sometimes to be based on an accidental connection between the emotional arousal and a particular place or situation. MacKinnon and Michels (1971) give the example of a man who took refuge in a movie theatre during a bombardment of his city and later developed an aversion to movies.

Some psychoanalytic investigators advocate paying careful attention to every aspect of the patient's description of his symptoms in order to understand their psychological significance. As examples, a patient who is afraid of crowds might mention that people could brush up against her, suggesting concern about sexual feelings. Another might speak of the discomfort of being alone among many strangers, suggesting anxiety over separation and threats to dependency gratification.

The analyst also often makes inferences from patient reports, although these interpretations are not usually shared with the patient early in treatment. For example, a patient reporting a fear of sexual assault may be considered to be unaware of her own sexual desires while projecting them onto unknown strangers. Similarly, a patient who fears he might faint in a restaurant and have to be carried out on a stretcher may lead the analyst to infer unconscious exhibitionistic impulses. This is an area of controversy, however, since what a psychoanalyst may consider as confirming material spontaneously coming from the patient may be viewed by others as ideas or feelings suggested to the patient and then reinforced by the analyst to confirm preexisting theories.

Psychoanalytic theory often implies that insightful exploration of the unconscious meaning of a phobic symptom should then allow the patient to reenter the phobic situation without becoming panicky. However, as Freud himself recognized, this was often not the case. He suggested that agoraphobics had to be pushed to reenter feared situations *before* they could overcome their phobias. In a paper on technique, he stated:

> . . . the various forms of disease treated by us cannot all be dealt with by the same techniques . . . a new kind of activity comes into question . . . the phobias have already made it necessary for us to go beyond our former limits. One can hardly master a phobia if one waits till the patient lets the analysis influence him to give it up. He will never in that case bring into the analysis the material indispensable for a convincing resolution of the phobia. One must proceed differently. Take the sample of agoraphobia; there are two classes of it, one mild, the other severe. Patients belonging to the first class suffer from anxiety when they go into the street by themselves, but they have not yet given up going out alone on that account; the others protect themselves from the anxiety by altogether ceasing to go about alone. With these last one succeeds only when one can induce them by the influence of the analysis to behave like phobic patients of the first class—that is, to go into the street and to struggle with their anxiety while they make the attempt. One starts, therefore, by moderating the phobia so far; and it is only when that has been achieved at the physician's demand that the associations and memories come into the patient's mind which enable the phobia to be resolved (Freud, 1955, pp. 165–166).

Freud assumed that, in pushing patients to enter feared situations, he was making unconscious material more accessible to scrutiny in the treatment situation. With this material available, patients could then be helped to understand that their avoidance and anxiety resulted from displacement of unacceptable sexual, dependent, and aggressive wishes. If this insight and understanding are sufficient, then the propensity to panic should disappear.

This treatment is in fact sometimes successful, perhaps because of the specific interpretative approach. It may also be, however, that the patient was successfully pushed to enter feared situations at a time when he was no longer having panic attacks and was only blocked by his anticipatory anxiety, which could be extinguished by the experience of not panicking. It may also be the case that a close relationship with a therapist reduces the vulnerability to panic attacks, which may stem from an abnormally low threshold to separation anxiety.

It gradually became clear, however, that psychodynamically based treatment efforts were often unsuccessful and that many agoraphobics continued to experience panic after years of psychoanalytic exploration of their phobic symptoms. For example, the psychoanalyst Edwardo Weiss (1964) observed that the prognosis in agoraphobia was often unfavorable; some patients had been analyzed for as long as ten or fifteen years with little or no improvement. Weinstock (1959), who reported follow-up data on a mixed group of forty-six phobic patients (agoraphobics were not specified) who had completed psychoanalysis, found that only six (13 percent) were symptom free. How is this to be understood?

The history of psychoanalysis is replete with attempts to grapple with issues such as this. Symptoms or behavior could be understood dynamically, yet the imparting of this understanding to the patient failed to result in significant improvement. The seemingly logical conclusion was a reformulation of the patient's dynamics, the bottom line of which was that he was sicker than had originally been perceived. A prominent example is the division of hysterics into hysterics and hysteroids or oedipal and preoedipal or genital and oral subtypes in an attempt to deal with the observation that some hysterics responded well to psychoanalysis, while others became more impaired.

The reformulation of agoraphobic dynamics to explain lack of response to an insight-oriented approach is seen in Ovesey's work (1966). He wrote that agoraphobics were:

> . . . immature, passive, easily frightened persons, who are markedly inhibited in both assertion and aggression. They have little confidence in their capacities to meet adult responsibilities, to satisfy their needs, and to insure their survival. In consequence, their predominant mode of psychological adaptation is through magical, infantile dependence upon stronger, authoritative parental figures (p. 42).

Having said that, he outlined a treatment approach that relies only in part on promoting psychological insight in the phobic patient. Rather, the main focus of his treatment effect was to get the agoraphobic to "enter into the phobic situation again and again until he reconditions a new response free from neurotic anxiety." Moreover, any activity on the part of the therapist that facilitated this process was acceptable, whether it was a psychodynamic explanation of the phobic mechanism, walking in the streets with the patient, making home visits, and advocating tranquilizers or a drink before an outing, or writing and signing a safe conduct pass for patients to use in a magical way while venturing forth into situations they fear.

What we have is a logical treatment approach based on an unproven premise: that the inability of agoraphobics to utilize interpretation and insight more profitably stemmed from their basic ego weakness, specifically, from their inability to give up magical dependence as the only way to satisfy their needs and safeguard their security. In this vein, the best that could be expected was a transference cure in which the patient used the therapist in a magical or highly dependent fashion. That an insight-oriented approach did not regularly work—because of an underlying, still-active biological vulnerability to panic that was not specifically connected to intrapsychic conflict—was not entertained as a possibility.

This is the crux of the matter. It is the realization of this underlying biological vulnerability to panic attacks, accompanied by the development of effective somatic treatments to block these terrifying experiences, that has revolutionized the treatment of agoraphobia.

What role then remains for the imparting of psychological insight in the treatment of agoraphobia? Our colleagues, Phillip Muskin and Abby Fyer (1980), have addressed this question in a review of the systematic treatment of fourteen agoraphobics. These investigators have identified three response patterns to treatment with tricyclic antidepressants in their agoraphobic sample. One group of patients showed a rapid response, with quick resolution of phobic behavior once adequately medicated, and required little additional support or urging. The second type of response was seen in patients who continue to have high anticipatory anxiety, that is, they did not trust the medication to block their panics. These patients could be pushed to reenter feared situations only with great difficulty and might in the end still refuse to attempt certain behaviors that were not necessary for their daily functioning.

The third group identified by Muskin and Fyer was one "in which the symptom complex had taken on significance as a resolution of an unconscious conflict in one of a variety of areas of life, including work, family, and social relationships." In these cases, insight-oriented psychotherapeutic work was considered necessary before any change in symptom patterns could take place. One example involved a patient whose panic symptoms and restricted behavior appeared to help her handle conflicts over competitive and aggressive impulses. Her fear of and avoidance of success could be denied, and her flight from promising jobs could be attributed to her anxiety symptoms. The investigators felt that these psychological reinforcers of anxiety symptoms and phobic avoidance had to be understood by the patient before she could give up her phobic behavior. An alternative explanation, however, is that what was involved was the diminishing of the "secondary gain" from the panic attacks.

One of us had recently treated a young man who presented with panic attacks and agoraphobia but refused medication. A two-year psychotherapeutic exploration of his fears of assertiveness, competitiveness, and full assumptions of adult male roles led to almost a complete remission of phobic behavior, as well as greatly improved marital functioning. When he terminated treatment his only residual phobia was a fear of out-of-town vacations. One is tempted to assert that helping this patient understand his unconscious conflicts led to amelioration of his panic attacks and agoraphobia. Again, however, one could argue that the panics remitted spontaneously or because of the patient's trust in the therapist, and that the main accomplishment of treatment was to get the patient to try the avoided activities again.

Therapists treating agoraphobic patients must also pay attention to the impact of patient improvement on the patient's social system. Muskin and Fyer (1980) also reported several cases in which patients or their partners feared abandonment should the patient become more independent. Milton and Hafner (1979) found that agoraphobic patients whose marriages were rated as unsatisfactory prior to behavior therapy were less likely to improve during treatment and more likely to relapse during follow-up than those patients with satisfactory marriages. The marriages of a number of patients also appeared to be adversely influenced by their symptomatic improvement. This was observed in marriages where the patients' symptoms maintained largely affectionless "compulsory" marriages. In some relationships the patients' symptoms allowed their spouses to deny their own problems. In both situations, patient improvement was perceived as a threat to marital homeostasis.

As several women in "compulsory" marriages overcame agoraphobic difficulties, their husbands became increasingly worried that their wives would really leave them. They reacted to this by undermining their wives' self-confidence, often in subtle ways, and by hindering their progress in overcoming their agoraphobia. We should add, however, that we have also seen cases in which the successful treatment of agoraphobia permitted long-overdue amicable divorces, desired for many other reasons.

How then are we to put all this material together?

What we suggest is the following: The most economical, efficacious treatment for spontaneous panic attacks with or without associated agoraphobic features is imipramine. Unless some strong contraindication or unwillingness exists, patients with spontaneous panic attacks should be given a trial of this drug. Some will be off and running toward improvement; others not. Of those who remain at the starting block, some will be found to be paralyzed by anticipatory anxiety, and a variety of techniques may be used to deal with this.

Some patients will continue to experience difficulty, even after such additional treatment, either specifically with anxiety or agoraphobic symptoms or with a variety of other difficulties that either predated the treatment or were unmasked by it. Some of these patients will require marital or family therapy. Others may demonstrate the classic psychodynamic conflicts described in the psychoanalytic literature on agoraphobia or other difficulties that could logically be treated with an insight-oriented approach.

One might still argue that even if an insight-oriented approach worked, it would still not demonstrate that the patient had been blocked by unconscious conflict but, rather, that such an approach was effective simply because it most closely fit the patient's preconceptions about an effective intervention and was therefore the most persuasive. While this question of the specificity or nonspecificity of curative factors in psychoanalytically oriented treatment is heuristically crucial from a theoretical perspective, in our stepwise, pragmatic approach to treatment it is not important to resolve.

We thus suggest a hierarchy of interventions, with two goals in mind. The first is to help each patient in the simplest and most efficient possible manner, that is, to attempt no more for the patient than is actually required by his condition. The second is to use and conceptualize these various treatment approaches as sieving or screening operations. Those who do not respond to the first approach have a more complicated or widespread dysfunction that requires something more in terms of treatment. These additional treatments would thus be brought to bear only when clinically indicated by lack of progress.

This approach toward concomitant psychotherapy for psychiatric conditions treated with drugs may have wide applicability. Most of our combined drug and psychotherapy trials treat patients with a given diagnosis with one of several possible combinations of drugs and psychotherapy and then assess outcome. Predictors of who actually does best with each treatment approach are usually determined retrospectively, if at all. What we suggest is to use simple drug treatment as a sieve, to see who responds fully and who requires further treatment.

Future research strategies may involve making judgments, in advance, as to who needs what type of psychotherapy, followed by assigning patients randomly to several different forms of treatment. This would test our hypothesized predictors as well as compare the efficacy of different forms of psychotherapy for a given condition.

In the meantime, however, our incremental strategy deals with patients with complex clinical phenomena. For some conditions, such as moderate nonendogenous depressions, one may want to employ a placebo sieve even before using an active drug. If drug treatment does not accomplish the desired goals, some will respond to supportive psychotherapeutic interventions aimed simply at overcoming the residual effects on self-esteem or self-concept of the primary illness—that is, continued demoralization in a person recovered from a depression or psychotic episode or anticipatory anxiety in a person who experienced panic attacks. Others will not respond to this and may require more interpretive treatment, either to overcome remaining barriers to resumption of full functioning or to work towards fuller functioning, be it interpersonal, vocational, or any other area.

This approach may offend some as too mechanistic, idealistic, impractical, or complex. However, we suggest that it points a way out of the morass of ideological bias as a basis for treatment selection. It also offers a practical, reliable, and scientifically sound basis for teasing apart the complexities of psychiatric disorders via comparative treatment trials.

References

Fink, M., Taylor, M.A., and Volavka, J. Anxiety precipitated by lactate. *New Eng. J. Med., 281:*1129, 1970.

Freud, S. An infantile neurosis and other works. In *The standard edition of the complete psychological works of Sigmund Freud.* London: Hogarth Press, Vol. 17: pp. 165–166, 1955.

Hand, I., LaMontagne, Y., and Marks, I.M. Group exposure (flooding) in vivo for agoraphobics. *Br. J. Psychiat., 124:*588–602, 1974.

Klein, D.F. Delineation of two drug-responsive anxiety syndromes. *Psychopharmacologia, 5:*397–408, 1964.

———, and Fink, M. Psychiatric reaction patterns to imipramine. *Amer. J. Psychiat., 119:*432–438, 1962.

MacKinnon, R.A., and Michels, R. *The psychiatric interview in clinical practice.* Philadelphia: W.B. Saunders, 1971.

Matthews, A.M., Johnston, D.W., Lancashire, M., et al. Imaginal flooding and exposure to real phobic situations: Treatment outcome with agoraphobic patients. *Br. J. Psychiat., 129:*362–371, 1976.

Milton, F., and Hafner, J. The outcome of behavior therapy for agoraphobia in relation to marital adjustment. *Arch. Gen. Psychiat., 36:*807–811, 1979.

Muskin, P., and Fyer, A. Unpublished data, 1980.

Ovesey, L. The phobic reaction: A psychodynamic basis for classification and treatment. In Goldman, G.S., and Shapiro, D., (Eds.) *Developments in psychoanalysis at Columbia University.* New York: Hafner, 1966, p. 42.

Pitts, F.N., Jr., and McClure, J.N., Jr. Lactate metabolism in anxiety neuroses. *New Eng. J. Med., 277:*1328–1336, 1967.

Weinstock, H. Phobias and their vicissitudes. *J. Amer. Psychoanal. Assoc., 7:*182–192, 1959.

Weiss E. *Agoraphobia in the light of ego psychology.* New York: Grune and Stratton, 1964; p. 64.

Zitrin, C. M., Klein, D.F., and Woerner, M.G. Behavior therapy, supportive psychotherapy, imipramine, and phobias. *Arch. Gen. Psychiat., 35:*307–316, 1978.

———. Treatment of agoraphobics with group exposure in vivo and imipramine. *Arch. Gen. Psychiat., 37:*63–72, 1980.

CHAPTER 11

An Overview of Combined Psychopharmacology and Psychotherapy: Summing Up and Critical Comments

Gerald J. Sarwer-Foner

I HAVE BEEN GIVEN THE TASK of presenting an overview of combined pharmacotherapy and psychotherapy (Sarwer-Foner, 1960B, 1960 C, and 1980) as well as that of offering a summary of constructively critical comments on the splendid material presented in the preceding chapters.

Some Introductory Comments

For Psychotherapy

By psychotherapy, I am referring to what a trained psychiatrist, a medical psychotherapist, does with a patient who needs these medical procedures. Thus the context is medical therapy—a trained physician treating a patient with an illness. The "sociologic state" of being ill is opened to a person by a physician examining the patient and making a diagnosis of illness. The physician then establishes with the patient a treatment plan which is individual, that is, specific for the particular disease situation of this patient, at this time, and in the individual's personal social context. The physician's choice of the type of psychotherapy needed for the particular disorder is part of the treatment plan.

For Pharmacotherapy

It is clear that pharmacotherapy is a "medical procedure"—medicines prescribed by a trained physician and monitored in terms of their total effects on the human organism. It is important to cite the problem this way, since the equality or inequality of the standards used for assessing or discussing these therapeutic procedures is one of the controversial issues that emerges in some of the papers presented in this symposium. Thus I am discussing combined psychotherapy and pharmacotherapy by the physician with a particular patient.

A psychiatrist can use one of these treatments, both of them, or choose to "split" them, sending the patient to another physician for psychotherapy (or in some circumstances to a properly trained psychotherapist who is not a physician) while administering the pharmacotherapy himself.

Split treatment is not the context of my remarks. New problems of treatment, both psychotherapeutic and pharmacotherapeutic, are produced by a therapeutic split—a split transference, in which important transference distortions may or may not come up and be adequately explored. Among the many problems in split therapy are the inability to link psychotherapeutic and pharmacotherapeutic events and their emotional significance, since two separate therapies are involved, and the tendency toward a gradation of therapies, in either the patient's or in both patient's and doctor's minds, as "first-class" or more important therapy versus "second-class" or less important therapy. There is all too often a split in communication patterns between the patient and his two doctors which reflects, in the transference, realities from the patient's family life. These communication patterns may then not be confronted in the treatment, such as when patient speaks to his mother about some problems but not to his father, while dealing with his father about other problems not mentioned to his mother. There are many other difficulties in split or separated treatment, but they cannot, because of space, be discussed here.

I will now summarize some of the principles of combined psychotherapy-pharmacotherapy, when carried out by a trained psychiatrist skilled in both procedures (Sarwer-Foner, 1955, 1956, 1957A and B; 1960A, B, C, and D; 1963, 1966, 1975, 1980, and 1981C).

Psychotherapy and Pharmacotherapy: General Principles

Psychotherapy is only conducted with patients who the physician feels (and the patient usually agrees) are able to participate in the procedure and will make significant efforts to master those problems which may be partially or totally uncontrolled at that moment, thus producing symptoms. At the start of therapy the patient often, but not always, sees himself as an active participant in the process. The doctor helps him develop this feeling. The doctor establishes and uses the therapeutic alliance that exists between doctor and patient for the purpose of securing access to the mastering of his problems. I have elsewhere commented on the differences between the classic doctor-patient relationship and a psychotherapeutic doctor-patient relationship. In the psychotherapeutic doctor-patient relationship, the patient with the help of the doctor does the work, not as in the classic doctor-patient relationship in which the doctor alone does the work and applies the treatment.

It is clear that one will not give pharmacotherapy to a patient unless one believes that the symptoms the patient presents and the disease process producing the symptoms *cannot be mastered or dealt with by the patient in psychotherapy at that moment in time or space.* If this assumption is not correct—if the patient can in fact, with the help of the physician, correct and master the intrapsychic problems causing the symptoms and the suffering—then the psychotropic medication (pharmacotherapy) is not really needed (Sarwer-Foner, 1960C and 1980). The author realizes that there are mixed states in which one can give the patient medication for "one part only of the problem," such as in insomnia, while carrying on psychotherapy for the other major difficulties.

One uses a "target symptom" approach (Freyhan, 1960) to pharmacotherapy here in the context of combined psychotherapeutic-pharmacotherapeutic treatment. In this target symptom approach, one gives adequate dosage of a psychotropic medication whose "standard clinical pharmacological profile of the drug" (Sarwer-Foner, 1957B, 1960A, 1960D, and 1963) will reliably strike at physiological symptoms one wishes to change. For example, in a hyperactive patient, one may wish to give a phenothiazine or lithium to reduce the energy going to the striated muscles and hence alter locomotor activity. One may wish to reduce the overall energy of the patient, thus reducing the impulse to act, one may wish to induce better sleep, or one may wish to increase the patient's inner feeling of outgoingness (such as with adequate dosage of tricyclic antidepressants). The typical pharmacological profile of the drug, when present in the patient, confronts him with the ego-integrative problem of whether he can, and of how he can, better master his symptoms or the life problems producing his symptoms. He is confronted by the fact that he has not, at that moment in time and space, mastered certain problems at all or has dealt with them in an inferior way without the drug, compared to an actual or potentially better mastery of these symptoms, with better integration of himself as a person, when the drug action is present.

Thus the patient may perceive the act of taking the medicine as proof that he cannot handle his symptoms or problems without it, at least at that moment in time or space (Sarwer-Foner, 1960A, 1960D, 1975; Shapiro, 1964; Sirala, 1963). Also the patient may be convinced that the doctor must feel and believe this as well, for he would not otherwise prescribe the drug. Too frequently the patient does not feel that he can discuss these perceptions with the physician, in case it would look as though he is criticizing or doubting the doctor.

Combining Psychotherapy and Chemotherapy

In our teaching of the supportive psychotherapeutic relationship with an acutely psychotic patient, the doctor would operate under the basic assumption that the patient is potentially capable of pulling himself together and of taking more responsibility for himself in the total sense. This includes the potential capacity to handle those aspects of functioning which, at the moment, may be totally out of control or seem to be out of control.

After exploring the need for it with the patient, the physician would explain the need for neuroleptic medication. The physician would also inform the patient of the importance of having the medication at appropriate times, that the medicine would only be prescribed during the time the patient actually needs it, and that, as soon as the patient is able to function properly and handle things without medication, the medicine will be withdrawn or changed. The stating of these premises sets up in the patient's mind a target for testing the doctor's reliability and steadiness. The patient will, in his own way, test whether the doctor "knows what he is talking about" in terms of the hoped-for improvement as well as indicate whether he is willing or able to collaborate with the physician in regard to these issues. If the patient is willing to work with the physician, especially with the issue of needing and taking the medication, even while acutely psychotic, the stage is set for a "bonding" or therapeutic alliance between them and for the patient's testing of the doctor's reliability, honesty, and steadiness. At the same time, the patient will be ready for internal testing of how he is, of how he can handle things better, and of how the doctor perceives him to be. During this time the doctor is doing reality testing and supportive psychotherapy with the patient. In this acute crisis-intervention phase of the early treatment of a psychosis, the fact that the doctor understands the patient enough to give the patient what is needed, while encouraging the patient's active collaboration in the process of improving, will help cement the beginning of a doctor/patient supportive, psychotherapeutic relationship (Ostow, 1960; Rappaport, 1978; Sarwer-Foner, 1977, 1979, and unpublished).

The doctor's attitude that the patient can say meaningful things and can potentially master large areas of his life allows the patient to verbalize his thoughts and feelings at the best level that he can manage and genuinely encourages him to try to speak meaningfully about his problems. Through his intervention, the physician helps the patient deal realistically with daily living and with the realities of thoughts and feelings. The better the physician understands conscious and unconscious processes, the better is he able to apply ego-supportive psychotherapeutic interventions to strengthen the reality orientation of and deal supportively with even psychotic material from the patient. Psychoanalytic training and skills are of definite advantage (Azima and Sarwer-Foner, 1961; Gottschalf, 1968; Horowitt, 1956; Lesse, 1956; Ostow, 1960; Rappaport, 1978; Sarwer-Foner and Ogle, 1955, 1956; Sarwer-Foner, 1957A and B; 1960A, B, and C; 1963; 1966).

The length of drug therapy is left as a variable but given the definite implication that, when the patient can get along without the drug, the drug will be stopped (Sarwer-Foner, 1979, 1980, unpublished). By that time many patients will have learned how to use the drug, either with the doctor's help or on their own. Should a patient again go out of control, both medicine and the doctor's relationship are available to him as needed.

For some patients, suffering from illness consisting of a state-bound consciousness, such as psychotic depresssions (Sarwer-Foner, 1966), most types of manic-depressive illness, certain schizo-affective schizophrenias, some acute fulminating, brief schizo-affective psychoses (bouffées délirantes), some acute catatonic stupors, and catatonic excitement states, all that relates to being ill belongs *only* to that state-bound consciousness—and all that relates to being well belongs to another, (different), state of being and consciousness. These illnesses are at their most complex in this regard; it is as though the psychotic state no longer exists for the patient when he leaves it. As in the perception of experiencing wakefulness and sleep, when one is awake, there is no sleep and, when one is asleep, there is no wakefulness. Similarly, when there is psychosis, there is no health; when there is health, there is no psychosis. Patients who have had this type of experience as a state of being and so feel this way about illness or health avoid anything connected to the sick state when they are "healthy." They do this because experiencing any part of the sick state can cause all of it to return, just as any part of being asleep can cause you to fall totally asleep. Therefore, patients who recover from the state-bound level of consciousness associated with the foregoing acute clinical psychoses want no part of the physician, the hospital, or anything that reminds them of illness when they are well (Sarwer-Foner, 1966). This includes all the things they did while they were ill and very often includes the medicines that they had to take and the psychotherapy or other procedures in which they participated, or to which they were subjected while ill.

From what I have said, it should be clear that I never believed that patients who had a psychotic episode needed to be on unremitting maintenance neuroleptic therapy for the rest of their lives. I always preferred these individualized, personal therapeutic regimes. In recent years the development of serious side effects, among them tardive or persistent dyskinesia, has done much to bring the need for time-related and time-controlled drug therapies into focus. As a result, many who previously favored ongoing maintenance therapy have adopted a more favorable consideration, a target-symptom (Freyhan, 1960), patient-physician, cooperation-oriented approach to chemotherapy. This in itself tends to introduce more elements of a psychotherapeutic nature, even for those physicians who are not interested in psychotherapy as such.

All that is known about transference patterns, the patient's responses to drug taking, patient-drug-physician interactions, and their indications is applicable here (Azima and Sarwer-Foner, 1961; Ostow, 1960; Sarwer-Foner and Kealey, 1981; Sarwer-Foner, unpublished; Shapiro, 1964; Sirala, 1963; Sosowsky, 1980; Uhlenhuth et al., 1966; Winkelman, 1960; Wittenborn and May, 1966; Wynn et al., 1978). Dealing with the counter-transference is of crucial importance here (Sarwer-Foner, 1957B and 1960B; Sarwer-Foner and Koranyi, 1960), particularly concerning the ways in which these patients' transference patterns automatically provoke counter-transference feelings in the physician—feelings which will reflect and repeat the very nature of the interpersonal, interfamilial trauma which existed in the patient's background.

Comments on Controversial Issues

Several basic issues of considerable controversy were raised in this book.

The issue of the therapeutic specificity of the psychotropic drugs arose; several matters of public policy, or influences on public policy, are linked to this (Sarwer-Foner, 1980, 1981A, and unpublished).

The Therapeutic Nonspecificity of the Neuroleptic Drugs

It is clear that each of the neuroleptic drugs has, in adequate clinical dosage, a specific *pharmacological* profile but that this characteristic pharmacologic effect is *not of itself curative of the disease state.* Given this fact, the target symptom approach (Sarwer-Foner and Ogle, 1955 and 1956) to using psychopharmacology, developed independently by Fritz Freyhan (1960) and my team in the early days of psychopharmacology, is preferable to an "antipsychotic drug action" approach. The antipsychotic drug approach has become prevalent, particularly in state hospital settings; it generally operates on a reductionalistic view of the patient which is presented by rating scale measures done by nursing staff, orderlies, or other ancillary workers.

In the antipsychotic drug approach, the emphasis is on the overall effects on the patient's psychosis over the length of the patient's hospitalization, on discharge, and during follow up. Important differences often exist between the standards for improvement, cure, and discharge of a patient from hospital used by state psychiatric hospitals and those used for nonpsychiatric general hospitals and general-hospital psychiatric units. The general-hospital psychiatric units often use the same criteria as those of the community as a whole for discharge into the community, that is, readiness to live in the community. This is similar to the standards which medical practice uses for the appropriate social behavior of "cured" or healthy patients. Rather than requiring similar criteria such as being "like the rest of the normal community," the state hospital is often forced to be satisfied with a patient who is no longer agitated or violent, who may be quietly hallucinating, as suitable for discharge.

Here are very important implications for public policy (Sarwer-Foner, 1980, 1981, in press). Among these is: *the therapeutic nonspecificity of our present neuroleptic drugs.* You can use *specific curative drugs* to treat diseases for which there are specific cures, such as using penicillin to combat penicillin-sensitive bacteria, without first understanding the psychodynamics of a patient's intrapsychic conflicts and life-crisis situation.

When one has a specific curative agent, adequate public policy may require a correct diagnosis and a proper application of the "cure"—the result is a cured patient. If there is a shortage of trained medical manpower, one could have a public policy of allowing nonmedical personnel to apply the treatment as long as a proper diagnosis has been made by a trained physician. This works easily for diseases in which medical auxiliaries can inject the curative antibiotic or the preventive vaccine. Here one teaches a specific procedure—injection or vaccination—to medical auxiliaries because one has a specific curative or preventative procedure.

We cannot, however, appropriately allocate as "good public policy" the treatment of major psychiatric illnesses for which we have no pharmacologic cure. Auxiliary personnel, lacking in training and medical techniques, cannot employ therapeutically nonspecific drugs; doing this would institute a version of "poor public-health policies" for psychiatric diseases.

Currently, in the treatment of schizophrenia, it behooves us to use all that is known about the psychodynamics, life stress, and social rehabilitative aspects of the disease, as well as the action of neuroleptics, since we do not have specific pharmacological curative agents. Furthermore, in the absence of specific curative agents, we cannot be indifferent to the task of training adequate numbers of psychiatrists to diagnose and treat these patients (Sarwer-Foner, 1980, 1981, and in press). Here there is a major and crucial public policy focus on training a large number of needed additional psychiatrists.

Public policy which responds to the social needs of schizophrenic patients. Does one keep patients as patients, that is, under medical control and aegis, or does one turn them over to a nonmedical social welfare ministry? If the latter, are poor hotels and flophouses better for these individuals' needs than are the average state hospitals? Can one have well-prepared, extramural, suitable housing with recreational facilities for discharged schizophrenic patients, as well as good rather than average mental hospitals for those who need long-term care? Is inferior or nonexistent community housing for these patients preferable to conditions in an average state hospital?

Public Policy of Control Clinical Trials to Prove Therapeutic Efficacy

For more than twenty-five years we have seen how social science rating instruments using statistical techniques (such as analysis of covariance) have progressed in assessing certain aspects of pharmacotherapy. Is this now equally applicable to psychotherapy? Certainly not in the same way. In the one-to-one psychotherapeutic relationship, there is the assumption that the patient will delve intrapsychically with the help of the physician. We ask that the patient look at his symbolizations, feelings, and thoughts in relationship to an intrapsychic image of himself, which includes his body image and his ego-defense mechanisms. In short, it includes a whole series of concepts that have been described naturalistically but have been confirmed by the combined experience of everyone who has used the same tools and the same general groups of techniques for approximately 100 years. Techniques appropriate for studying this process will have to be evolved; they cannot be simply assumed reductionalistically, borrowed from social science statistics.

Similarly, in Mr. Hogarty's chapter, in the discussion of sociotherapy (social manipulation, manipulation of external environmental factors, attempts oriented to help the patient develop better mastery of specific areas of life situations), he gives good anecdotal material and clear descriptions offering a picture of what he is discussing. Would these descriptions stand up to the rigors of imposed clinical testing, would they replicate if someone else repeated the work using the same data and the same criteria with different sets of patients? Would the latter allow a measurable record? Most of us hope that it would (Goldberg et al., 1977; Hogarty et al., 1974; Horowitt, 1956). Some might say that one has to use a social science reductionalistic rating scale, a brief psychiatric rating scale, or similar, which could be measured statistically—or they wouldn't accept the data. I think that many of us would disagree with this point of view, not because we are against statistics in science, but because the statistics used must be appropriate to the total phenomenon being measured, not merely a reductionalistic measure of only part of the phenomenon which is then treated as though it were the whole. In short, if we are talking about controlled clinical trials, we should be talking about well-designed, appropriate, psychotherapeutic ones.

Dr. Goodwin has given an elegant description of his patient, who indicated that "the drug made me controllable, made me relate, made me carry on but it is the psychotherapeutic interaction that allows me to feel that I am mastering that which up until then was not mastered." Here I can use both his work and mine (Sarwer-Foner, 1966) to illustrate an aspect of the combined use of psychotherapy and psychopharmacology with psychotic patients whose diseases with state-bound consciousness respond well to psychotropic drugs. These drugs work well on the condition that (1) the clinical psychopharmacological profile of the drug is present, (2) the drug is being given in adequate dosage, and (3) the presence of this clinical psychopharmacological profile controls symptom complexes of importance to the patient. The control of these symptom complexes has to signify for the particular patient a newly acquired mastery or partial mastery over the core of his problems, which he could not master at this moment without the drug effect. If these conditions are met, the patient begins to feel more internally secure. The patient then tests whether his perception of relative internal change is shared by significant people of his environment. The patient is very sensitive and has low self-esteem, particularly when he feels out of control in his psychosis. Thus, even if he feels relatively changed for the better internally, he has to compare his view of the change with those of his significant relationships. If his entourage of significant people reinforces the patient's view that he has indeed changed, then he continues to integrate. If his entourage denies the patient's internal view of having changed for the better, then the neuroleptic effect is generally not enduring, and the patient relapses or his condition worsens, even though the drug effect is present.

Mr. Hogarty has referred to both the work of Professor Wing in

England and some of his own data; and in a different context, you read Myrna Weissman's description of what helps people feel that they are doing well or, conversely, breaking down. If you expose a patient who is recovering from a psychosis to a highly involved, emotional, rejecting family, the patient often will feel unaccepted by them, misunderstood, and overly criticized. A patient usually breaks down remarkably rapidly in the face of these conditions. If there is a more neutral setting in which the patient can be encouraged to master aspects of social living, new skills, and so on then the medication, when properly given to the right patient, helps him do this, and the sociological, rehabilitative results seem better.

Trained clinicians who know schizophrenia—its clinical nature, its psychodynamic structure, the way the patient behaves—know that schizophrenic patients attempt to minimize their own pain and use their character defenses and often their resulting life-style in this direction. They monitor the physicians carefully in this regard, keeping us away from the areas of danger or pain that they cannot stand. Lewis Hill (1957) said years ago that schizophrenia is a way of life, alluding to these proclivities in the patient, and many professionals, including Otto Will, would today agree.

If, as a matter of public policy, one decides to close asylums and modern hospitals that attend the chronically ill (or those which offer some aspects of long-term hospitalization for schizophrenia, including good [two-to-five year] rehabilitative programs which improve prognosis for leaving the hospital) and have patients live "only" in the community, then certain events are going to occur. One should not interpret my remarks to mean that I am against rehabilitating patients into the community; I believe that all patients who can improve sufficiently to live adequately in the community are far better off than they might be while living in a state or chronic hospital. Patients—for whom adequate community resources do not exist and for whom the type of care and nurturing that a good hospital program supplies is necessary—will suffer the results of the undifferentiated public policy of attempting to close hospitals which offer long-term mental care; these patients will be thrown into an unprepared and unreceptive community (*Life,* 1981). The procedures used by some states to "treat" schizophrenic patients are far from ideal; practices may include throwing them into the community, even if a mental health center is made responsible for them, or depending on as few as four days of hospitalization with follow-up social rehabilitation programs. The point is, would you or I individualize the treatment of each patient or choose this type of treatment? In states with minimal resources or negative public policy, it is important to analyze the conditions under which patients are arrested and detained in jail and how long they are detained, compared to how long they would stay in a hospital. Public policy as it relates to helpless, voiceless, and politically powerless patients is a very large issue indeed—and a largely unsolved one.

Is there to be little or no money for training adequate numbers of psychiatrists, little or no money for rehabilitation into the community, or for proper intrahospital care in good, long-term hospitals with good rehabilitative programs? By funding limited resources to psychiatry, one can play the "poor public-health approach" to treating schizophrenic patients. Proper public policy in relationship to the major psychoses would include a realistic assessment of the presently available therapies, a realization that we must have enough properly trained psychiatrists to use all our present psychiatric armature—psychotherapy, sociotherapy, and pharmacotherapy. The more difficult patients will best respond to any one, or any combination, of all of these, and only a skilled psychiatrist responsible for a particular patient can best determine the patient's needs.

Another issue, raised specifically by Dr. Klerman in his comments, is the one of controlled clinical trials to prove the efficacy of a treatment. No one can do other than agree in principle that this is a good policy, but there are many *buts.* For such a policy to be properly applied, the criteria for what tools are appropriate to best assess a particular therapeutic procedure have to be carefully defined. Reductionalistic rating scale techniques are at best "witnesses" (in the religious sense of "bearing testimonial") to only selected therapeutic processes.

Careful case description, with description of psychotherapeutic techniques, treatment plan, and criteria for what we hope to change and for assessment of such changes, can be the valid procedure to link what has been reported in the psychoanalytic and psychotherapeutic literature over the past 100 years. Confirmation of case findings by others, over time, offers a reasonable way of assessing and documenting both the past successes with a particular technique and its comparison with those techniques currently in use.

If public policy demands specialized clinical assessment of the efficacy of psychotherapy, then discussions with real experts in the field would first have to define which techniques of treatment are appropriate to the procedures; shall we use reductionalistic rating scales, reviews of simple video tapes, particular sessions in audiotapes, or what other means?

In short, it is not the concept of controlled clinical trials that is controversial; rather, it is some of the doubts about which central policy measures will really produce an appropriate, unprejudiced assessment of psychotherapy, psychoanalysis, and other such procedures that is the issue.

For example, Mr. Hogarty's sociotherapy—monthly contact with a social worker to deal with issues of living in the community—for a residual schizophrenic patient cannot be characterized as psychotherapy if strict assessment criteria for psychotherapy are applied. If we attempt to analyze covariance, then a great deal of statistical planning and testing will have to occur before we can agree that these largely reductionalistic techniques are appropriate in the assessment of psychotherapy.

I cannot agree with a public policy, such as exists in some jurisdictions, of having only four days of hospitalization for an acute recrudescence of a schizophrenic patient who was previously neuroleptically treated. All the study and analysis of the data related to keeping patients out of the hospital with such an approach only provides information about what four days of hospitalization permits. It suggests nothing about what is the best way, or the proper way, to treat acute schizophrenic exacerbations; it completely neglects consideration of what might be the very best course of therapy for an individual schizophrenic patient if the entire normal gamut of therapies were available for the treatment of such a patient.

References

AZIMA, H., and SARWER-FONER, G.J. Psychoanalytic formulations of drugs in pharmacotherapy. *Rev. Can. Biol.*, June *20*:603, 1961.

FREYHAN, F. Neuroleptic effect: Fact or fiction. In Sarwer-Foner, G.J. (Ed.), *The dynamics of psychiatric drug therapy*. Springfield, Ill.: Charles C Thomas, 1960.

GOLDBERG, S.C., SCHOOLER, N.R., HOGARTY, G.E., and ROPER, M. Prediction of relapse in schizophrenic outpatients treated by drug and sociotherapy. *Arch. Gen. Psychiat.*, 34:171, 1977.

GOTTSCHALT, L.A. Some problems in the use of psychoactive drugs, with or without psychotherapy, in the treatment of non-personality disorders. In

Efron, D.H. (Ed.), *Psychopharmacology: A review of process, 1957–1967.* Washington, D.C.: Public Health Service Publication No. 1836, 1968; p. 225.

Hill, L.B. The nature of extramural schizophrenia. In Rifkin, A.H., (Ed.), *Schizophrenia in psychoanalytic office practice.* New York: Grune and Stratton, 1957.

Hogarty, G.E., Goldberg, S.C., Schooler, M.R., et al. Drug and sociotherapy in the aftercare of schizophrenic patients II. Two year relapse rates. *Arch. Gen. Psychiat.*, 31:603, 1974.

Horowitt, K.F. Fact and artifact in the biology of schizophrenia. *Science,* 124:3219, 1956.

Lesse, S. Psychotherapy and ataractics: Some observations on combined psychotherapy and chlorpromazine therapy. *Amer. J. Psychother., 10*:448, 1956.

Life Magazine. Emptying the madhouse. May 1981, 56–70.

Ostow, M. The use of drugs to overcome technical difficulties in psychoanalysis. In Sarwer-Foner, G.J. (Ed.), *Dynamics of Psychiatric Drug Therapy.* Springfield, Ill.: Charles C Thomas, 1960; pp. 443–463.

Rappaport, M. Are drugs more than palliative in the management of schizophrenia? In Brady, J.P., and Brodie, H.K.H., (Eds.), *Controversy in psychiatry.* Philadelphia: Saunders, 1978; pp. 205–232.

Sarwer-Foner, G.J. Psychoanalytic theories of activity-passivity conflicts and the continuum of ego defenses. Experimental verification with reserpine and chlorpromazine. *Arch. Neurol. Psychiat., 78:*413, 1957. (A)

———. The transference and the nonspecific drug effects in the use of the tranquilizing drugs and their influence on affect. *Psych. Research Report,* 1957, *8:*153–167. (B)

———. *The dynamics of psychiatric drug therapy.* Springfield, Ill.: Charles C Thomas, 1960. (A)

———. Some therapeutic aspects of the use of neuroleptic drugs in schizophrenic, borderline states and in short-term psychotherapy of the neuroses. In Sarwer-Foner, G.J., (Ed.), *Dynamics of psychiatric drug therapy.* Springfield, Ill.: Charles C Thomas, 1960; p. 517. (B)

———. The role of the neuroleptic medication in psychotherapeutic interaction. *Comp. Psych., 1:*291–300, 1960. (C)

———. On the mechanisms of action of neuroleptic drugs: A theoretical psychodynamic explanation. Hassan Azima Memorial Lecture, in Wortis, J., (Ed.), *Recent advances in biological psychiatry,* Vol. VI. New York: Plenum Press, 1963; pp. 217–232.

———. A psychoanalytic note on a specific delusion of time in psychotic depressions. *Can. Psychiat. Assc. Journ. Suppl., 11:*S221, 1966.

———. On psychiatric symptomatology: Its meaning and function in relation to the psychodynamic actions of drugs. In Denber, H.C.B., (Ed.), *Psychopharmacological treatment in psychiatry.* New York: Marcel Dekker, 1975.

———. An approach to the global treatment of the borderline patient: Psychoanalytic, psychotherapeutic, and psychopharmacological consideration. In Horticollis, P., (Ed.), *Borderline personality disorders.* New York: International Universities Press, 1977.

———. Comments on antipsychotics vs. specific therapy. In Denber, H.C.B., (Ed.), *Schizophrenia: Theory, diagnosis, and treatment.* New York: Marcel Dekker, 1979; pp. 179–221.

———. *Combined psychotherapy and pharmacotherapy in specialized techniques in individual psychotherapy.* Karasu, T., and Bellack, L. (Eds.), New York: Brunner/Mazel, 1980.

———. *Schizophrenia 1980: Implications for psychopharmacology in psychiatry, psychopharmacology, and alternatives: Trends for the 80's.* Schwab, J. (Ed.), New York: Marcel Dekker, 1981. (A)

———. Philosophy of quality care, role modeling of residents, and the organization of quality services. Read at the American Psychiatric Association Symposium: Quality of Care Delivery by Teaching Hospitals, May 5, 1980, San Francisco, Calif. *Psychiatric Journ. Univ. Ottawa, 6:*4–12, 1981.

———. Some thought on the current status of the schizophrenic group of illnesses: Treatment, research, and social aspects. The Simon Bolivar Lecture, 134th Annual Meeting of American Psychiatric Association, Grand Ballroom, Hilton Hotel, New Orleans, Thursday, May 14, 1981. To be published.

———. and KEALEY, L.S. Reactions to hospitalization: Passive dependency factors. Recurrence of original symptoms and attempts to prolong hospitalization on the announcement of discharge. *Comp. Psychiat., 22:*1:103–133, 1981.

———. and KORANYI, E.K. Transference effects, the attitude of the treating physician, and countertransference in the use of neuroleptic drugs. In Sarwer-Foner, G.J., (Ed.), *Dynamics of psychiatric drug therapy.* Springfield, Ill.: Charles C Thomas, 1960.

———. and OGLE, W. Use of reserpine in open psychiatric settings. *Can. Med. Assoc. J., 73:*187, 1955.

———. Psychosis and enhanced anxiety produced by reserpine and chlorpromazine. *Can. Med. Assoc. J., 74:*526, 1956.

SHAPIRO, A.K. Etiological factors in placebo effect. *J. Amer. Med. Assoc., 1964,* 187:712.

SIRALA, M. Schizophrenia: A human situation. *Amer. J. Psychoanal., 23:*39–58, 1963.

SOSOWSKY, L. Explaining the increased arrest rate among mental patients: A cautionary note. *Amer. J. Psychiat., 137:*1602–1605, 1980.

UHLENHUTH, E.M., RICKELS, K., FISHER, S., PARK, L.C., LIPMAN, R.S., and Mock J. Drug, doctor's verbal attitude, and clinical setting in the symptomatic response to pharmacotherapy. *Psychopharmacologia* (Berlin), *9:*392, 1966.

WINKLELMAN, N.W., JR. Chlorpromazine and prochlorperazine during psychoanalytic psychotherapy. In Sarwer-Foner, G.J., (Ed.), *Dynamics of psychiatric drug therapy.* Springfield, Ill.: Charles C Thomas, 1960, p. 134.

WITTENBORN, J.R., and MAY, P.R.A. *Prediction of Response to Pharmacotherapy.* Springfield, Ill.: Charles C Thomas, 1966.

WYNN, L.C., CROMWELL, R.L., and MATTHYSSE, S., (EDS.), *The nature of schizophrenia: New approaches to research and treatment.* New York: Wiley Medical, 1978.

Index